A Colour Atlas of

OBESITY

Dr Roland T. Jung

MA, MD(Cantab), FRCP, FRCP(Ed).

*Consultant Physician with specialist interest in
Obesity, Endocrinology and Diabetes Mellitus
Honorary Senior Lecturer in
Department of Medicine*

*Ninewells Hospital and Medical School
Dundee, Scotland*

Wolfe Medical Publications Ltd

Copyright © Roland T. Jung, 1990
Published by Wolfe Medical Publications Ltd, 1990
Printed by Grafos, Arte Sobre Papel, Barcelona, Spain
ISBN 0 7234 1577 3

A CIP catalogue record for this book is available from the British Library.

This book is one of the titles in the series of Wolfe Medical Atlases, a
series that brings together the world's largest systematic published
collection of diagnostic colour photographs.

For a full list of Wolfe Medical Atlases, plus forthcoming titles and details
of our surgical, dental and veterinary Atlases, please write to Wolfe
Medical Publications Ltd, 2-16 Torrington Place, London WC1E 7LT
England.

Contents

Preface

'How boring, yet another obese patient' was the overheard comment. How untrue. The obese patient presents one of the most perplexing challenges which modern science is only now beginning to investigate in depth. The mortality and morbidity of this condition makes it one of the most important nutritional problems of modern society with a high financial cost. There is much diverse interest in this subject from the basic research done on animals to human experimentation, epidemiological studies, clinical management of the morbid sequelae, treatment and prevention. This involves many specialities of medicine and science each with their own specialised journals, textbooks and approach.

The aim of this Atlas is to represent a broad visual spectrum of obesity, giving brief descriptions where necessary but not going into any one subject in too great a depth. Where a few references are useful they are included but this book is mainly designed to be a visual reference in itself. I hope that I have covered most aspects of obesity, sufficiently illustrated, to satisfy the expert but more importantly to whet the appetite of the newcomer whether they be a student, a research scientist, dietician, nutritionalist, nurse or clinician, any person in fact with a positive interest in obesity. Hopefully more will realise that obesity is anything but boring.

Although every effort has been made to check for accuracy the author and publishers advise that diagnosis and treatment should never be made or instituted on the material contained within this book alone.

Dr Roland T. Jung
Department of Medicine
Ninewells Hospital and Medical School
Dundee, Scotland

Acknowledgements

In the preparation of this Atlas I received the general assistance of many of my colleagues without which this book would never have been completed. I would especially like to thank the following who allowed publication of pictures from their collections:

Professor G.F. Joplin, Dr J.W. Shaw, Dr D.A. Price, Dr A.S. McCullough, Dr C.C. Forsyth, Mr A.M. Morris, Professor C. Forbes, Dr W. Guthrie, Dr J. Belch, Mr N. Fowkes, Dr R. Newton, Dr N.J. Douglas, Mr A. Gunn, Dr P. Mitchell, Mr P. Preece, Dr D. Walsh, Professor W.P.T. James, Dr J. Doran, Dr R.G. Whitehead, Mr I. Duncan, Dr J. Gregory, Mr J. Mills, Dr G. Lowe, Dr G. McNeil, Dr K. Kenicer, Mr N. Kennedy, Mr P. Baines, Dr C. Paterson, Dr B.M. Laurance. Dr M. Kerr, Dr D.C.L. Savage, Professor J. Lever, Dr J.A. Thomson, Dr I.W. Campbell, Professor R.L. Himsworth, Dr S. Morley, Professor C.R.W. Edwards, Dr G. Howie, Dr R. MacWalter, Dr I. Henderson, Dr N.W. Oakley, Dr K.A. Hussein, Dr C. Kelner, Dr J. Coleiro, Dr M. White, Dr M. Boulton-Jones and Dr N. Peden.

My thanks also to the patients who gave permission for their clinical pictures to be shown, and to the many editors and publishers who allowed me to republish data, figures and tables already published elsewhere. Each is referenced in the text and acknowledged in the following section. I also thank Ms M. Hughes for typing both the extensive correspondence and the manuscript. Finally, and most importantly, my special gratitude goes to Mr King and his staff in the Medical Illustration Department at Ninewells Hospital, Dundee, for their skilled photography and preparation of the many clinical pictures.

Acknowledgements for Published Material

Table 1, Table 2, 212 Reproduced courtesy of Editor, Journal of Royal College of Physicians of London and Professor W.P.T. James, Secretary to the Working Party on Obesity for the report (ref. 1).

7 Reproduced courtesy of Professor J. Garrow and Editor, Annals of Human Biology for Taylor and Francis Ltd. (ref. 2 and 3).

Table 5 Reproduced courtesy of the Editor, British Journal of Nutrition and Cambridge University Press (ref. 4).

15 Detailed charts are available from Castlemead Publications, Hertford, U.K.

26 Reprinted with permission from The New England Journal of Medicine, 314, 195, 1986 (ref. 5).

28 Reproduced courtesy of Professor W.P.T. James and Editor, Lancet (ref. 6).

29 Reprinted with permission from The New England Journal of Medicine, 318, 465, 1988 (ref. 9).

30 Reprinted with permission from The New England Journal of Medicine 318, 496, 1988 (ref. 11).

40 Reproduced courtesy of Editor, Anatomical Record, publication of Wistar Press (ref. 14).

51, 52, 53 Reproduced courtesy of Editor, British Medical Journal (ref. 18).

62, 63, 67, 68 Reproduced courtesy of Professor R. Himsworth, Dr C.J. Hawkey and Editor, Journal of Medical Genetics (ref. 21).

77 Reproduced with permission of Professor C. Chanter of Guy's Hospital, London. Plate copies courtesy of Butterworth Scientific from 12th Edition French's Index of Differential Diagnosis, Fig. 526, 1985.

88 Reproduced by permission from An Atlas of Characteristic Syndromes. A Visual Aid to Diagnosis. Wiedemann, Grosse, Dibbern (Ed). Wolfe Medical Publications, 1985. First published in ref. 23.

152, 153, 154, 155, 156 Reproduced courtesy of Dr R. Newton and MTP Press (ref. 24).

182, 183 Courtesy of Dr R. Turner, Radcliffe Infirmary, Oxford.

194, 195, 196 Reproduced courtesy of Editor, Hospital Update (ref. 26), Dr M.C. White Dr F. White, Professor C.W. Home and Dr. B. Angus.

224, 326 Reproduced courtesy of U.S. Department of Health, Education and Welfare (ref. 28).

225 Reprinted with permission from The New England Journal of Medicine, 304, 932, 1981 (ref. 29).

251 Reproduced courtesy of Editor, The Practitioner (ref. 30).

247, 248, 249, 250 Courtesy of Professor C. Forbes, Dr J. Belch and J.H. McKillop.

313, 314 Reproduced courtesy of Editor, Update (ref. 33).

369 Reprinted with permission from The New England Journal of Medicine, 284, 1237, 1971 (ref. 42).

370, 371 Reprinted with permission from The New England Journal of Medicine, 311, 1405, 1406, 1984 (ref. 43).

372 Reproduced courtesy of Editor, International Journal of Obesity (ref. 44).

374 Reproduced courtesy of Editor, Lancet (ref. 46).

375 Reproduced courtesy of Dr P. Kopelman and Editor, Clinical Endocrinology, Blackwell Scientific Publications Ltd. (ref. 47).

451, 452, 453 Reproduced courtesy of the Editor, Lancet (ref. 53).

458 Cord and button, courtesy of Dr J. Munro, Edinburgh.

460 Reproduced courtesy of Editor, British Medical Journal (ref. 58).

468 Reproduced courtesy of Mr T.V. Taylor and Dunlop Limited, Precision Rubber Division.

Dedication

To my little daughter who regularly visited my study (and emptied my bookshelves) during the preparation of this work.

1 Assessment of Obesity

1 Beam balance is necessary for accurate measurement of weight. This instrument is strong, portable and accurate. Babies can also be measured as the cradle can be separately weighed.

2 Sitting scales are only useful for mildly overweight patients as many obese patients do not fit in the chair.

3 Conventional scales may weigh up to 165 kg but for very obese subjects the platform is too small, the abdomen or bottom limiting patients' ability to stand on the platform unaided. The height stick is useless for any accurate measurement.

4 250 kg Top Limit Scales. This model has a wide platform to accommodate a large abdomen and also has a dial for easy reading.

5 A stadiometer is used for accurate measurement of height, essential for children. It is important that the technique used is precise. The child stands on a flat surface, usually the floor, with his back to the stadiometer. Shoes and socks are removed and heels touch the steel backboard. Legs should be straight with buttocks and scapulae touching the backplate of the device. As heads vary in shape a standard position of the skull is used, namely that the lower margins of the orbit are in the same horizontal plane as the external auditory meati. Upward pressure is then applied below the mastoids to lift the head and eliminate postural changes. Then the platform is lowered to rest on the head and the measurement made while the child has exhaled.

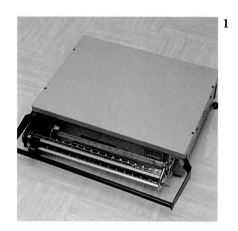

1

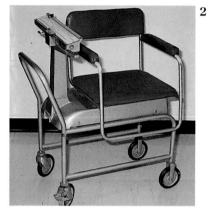

2

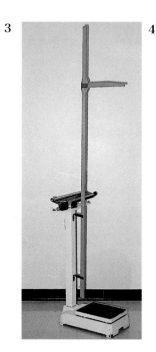

3

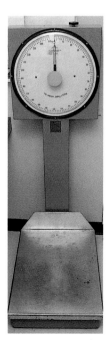

4

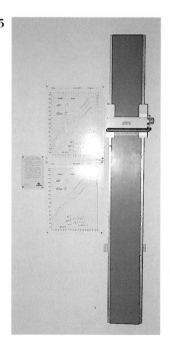

5

Table 1. Guidelines for body weight in adults

Metric

Height without shoes (m)	Men Weight without clothes (kg)			Women Weight without clothes (kg)		
	Acceptable average	Acceptable weight range	Obese	Acceptable average	Acceptable weight range	Obese
1.45				46.0	42-53	64
1.48				46.5	42-54	65
1.50				47.0	43-55	66
1.52				48.5	44-57	68
1.54				49.5	44-58	70
1.56				50.4	45-58	70
1.58	55.8	51-64	77	51.3	46-59	71
1.60	57.6	52-65	78	52.6	48-61	73
1.62	58.6	53-66	79	54.0	49-62	74
1.64	59.6	54-67	80	55.4	50-64	77
1.66	60.6	55-69	83	56.8	51-65	78
1.68	61.7	56-71	85	58.1	52-66	79
1.70	63.5	58-73	88	60.0	53-67	80
1.72	65.0	59-74	89	61.3	55-69	83
1.74	66.5	60-75	90	62.6	56-70	84
1.76	68.0	62-77	92	64.0	58-72	86
1.78	69.4	64-79	95	65.3	59-74	89
1.80	71.0	65-80	96			
1.82	72.6	66-82	98			
1.84	74.2	67-84	101			
1.86	75.8	69-86	103			
1.88	77.6	71-88	106			
1.90	79.3	73-90	108			
1.92	81.0	75-93	112			
BMI	22.0	20.1-25.0	30.0	20.8	18.7-23.8	28.6

Non-metric

Height without shoes (ft. in)	Men Weight without clothes (lb)			Women Weight without clothes (lb)		
	Acceptable average	Acceptable weight range	Obese	Acceptable average	Acceptable weight range	Obese
4 10				102	92-119	143
4 11				104	94-122	146
5 0				107	96-125	150
5 1				110	99-128	154
5 2	123	112-141	169	113	102-131	152
5 3	127	115-144	173	116	105-134	161
5 4	130	118-148	178	120	108-138	166
5 5	133	121-152	182	123	111-142	170
5 6	136	124-156	187	128	114-146	175
5 7	140	128-161	193	132	118-150	180
5 8	145	132-166	199	136	122-154	185
5 9	149	136-170	204	140	126-158	190
5 10	153	140-174	209	144	130-163	196
5 11	158	144-179	215	148	134-168	202
6 0	162	148-184	221	152	138-173	208
6 1	166	152-189	227			
6 2	171	156-194	233			
6 3	176	160-199	239			
6 4	181	164-204	245			

Table 1 Guidelines for body weight in adults
Based on the Metropolitan Life Insurance tables and
published by the Royal College of Physicians of London.
Metric and nonmetric guidelines are illustrated. Note that
frame size is no longer shown as it is difficult to estimate
someone's frame size. The acceptable weight range for
each height group, therefore, encompasses all frame sizes.
Overweight is defined as when an individual exceeds the
upper limit of the full range of weights for his/her height and
obesity is defined as a weight of 120% or more above the
upper limit (itself defined as 100%) of the acceptable range
(ref. 1).

Table 2 Guidelines for body weight in children
Published by the Royal College of Physicians of London and
based on the USA Health and Nutritional Examination
Survey of 1971-1974. Children who exceed the 97th centile
weight for height are considered overweight. These figures
are based on the average weight of children in a well
nourished society, not on morbidity or mortality risk as in
adults (ref. 1).

Table 2. Guidelines for body weight in children

BOYS

Percentile	3rd	50th	97th	3rd	50th	97th
Age (yr)		Stature (cm)			Weight (kg) at median height	
2.0	79.6	85.6	91.6	10.2	12.2	14.9
2.5	83.8	90.4	97.0	11.1	13.3	16.1
3.0	87.8	94.9	102.1	12.0	14.4	17.3
3.5	91.5	99.1	106.7	12.9	15.4	18.5
4.0	94.9	102.9	111.0	13.8	16.5	19.7
4.5	98.2	106.6	114.9	14.7	17.6	20.8
5.0	101.3	109.9	118.6	15.7	18.7	22.0
5.5	104.2	113.1	122.0	16.6	19.7	23.2
6.0	107.0	116.1	125.2	17.5	20.7	24.6
6.5	109.6	119.0	128.3	18.5	21.9	26.1
7.0	112.1	121.7	131.3	19.3	22.8	27.5
7.5	114.5	124.4	134.2	20.4	24.1	29.5
8.0	116.9	127.0	137.0	21.4	25.2	31.2
8.5	119.2	129.6	139.9	22.4	26.5	33.1
9.0	121.5	132.2	142.8	23.4	27.8	35.2
9.5	123.8	134.8	145.9	24.7	29.6	37.8
10.0	126.0	137.5	149.0	25.8	31.2	40.2

GIRLS

Percentile	3rd	50th	97th	3rd	50th	97th
Age (yr)		Stature (cm)			Weight (kg) at median height	
2.0	78.5	84.4	90.4	9.7	11.7	14.2
2.5	82.9	89.5	96.1	10.5	12.6	15.3
3.0	86.9	94.0	101.0	11.5	13.8	16.8
3.5	90.6	97.9	105.3	12.4	14.9	18.0
4.0	94.0	101.6	109.1	13.2	15.8	19.0
4.5	97.5	105.0	112.9	14.0	16.8	20.1
5.0	100.1	108.4	116.7	14.8	17.8	21.3
5.5	102.8	111.6	120.3	15.6	18.7	22.4
6.0	105.4	114.6	123.9	16.5	19.7	23.7
6.5	107.9	117.6	127.4	17.5	20.8	25.2
7.0	110.3	120.6	130.9	18.5	22.0	27.0
7.5	112.3	123.0	133.8	19.4	23.1	28.6
8.0	115.0	126.4	137.7	20.7	24.8	31.4
8.5	117.5	129.3	141.1	21.9	26.5	34.1
9.0	120.0	132.2	144.5	23.0	28.0	36.7
9.5	122.6	135.2	147.8	24.4	30.1	40.3

Table 3. Quetelet Index	
Titian figure	25
Boticelli's Venus	23
Pin up Calender Model	22
Skinny Type Model	18
Sprint Athletic Olympic Champion, male	23
Marathon Champion, female	19

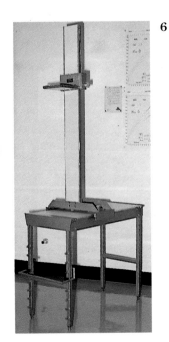

6

Table 3 Quetelet's index or body mass index (BMI)
Often used to express the degree of obesity. This index is
calculated from the equation weight (in kg) divided by the
square of the height (ht^2) measured in metres. A BMI of 30
or more in males, or 28.6 or more in females would be
indicative of obesity.

6 The sitting stadiometer is helpful to measure sitting
height accurately, especially useful in the assessment of
short and dysmorphic children.

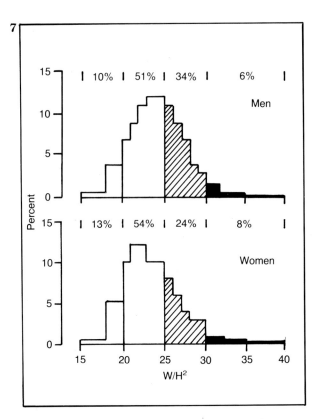

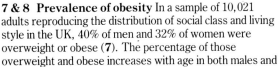

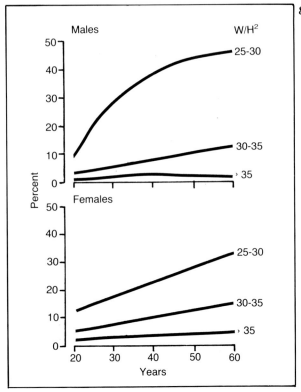

7 & 8 Prevalence of obesity In a sample of 10,021
adults reproducing the distribution of social class and living
style in the UK, 40% of men and 32% of women were
overweight or obese (**7**). The percentage of those
overweight and obese increases with age in both males and
females (**8**). The corresponding figures for the USA are
43% of males and 36% of females and for Australia, 41% of
males and 31% of females are overweight or obese (ref. 2
and 3).

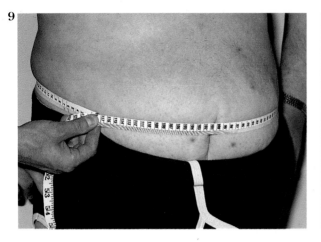
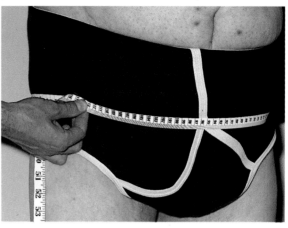

9 & 10 Regional fat distribution Comparison of the circumference of waist and hip is often measured. The circumference is measured around the waist in the erect position. Some measure at the umbilicus (**9**), others at a point one-third the distance between the xiphoid process and umbilicus. This measurement can be difficult in the very obese with large abdominal obesity. The hip circumference (**10**) is measured 4 cm below the superior iliac spine (without pants). Others advocate measuring the hip at a point one-third of the distance between the superior iliac spine and the patella. The importance of these measurements appears to be that those who deposit their fat abdominally rather than on their hips are particularly susceptible to cardiovascular disease and diabetes mellitus. In this respect a ratio of abdominal to hip girth of over 0.8 is considered hazardous.

Table 4. Body Composition	Weight (kg)	
Component	Normal weight male	Obese male
Water	42.0	51.4
Protein	13.0	16.0
Fat	11.0	48.6
Glycogen	0.5	0.5
Other	3.5	3.5
Total	70.0	120.0

Table 4 Body composition of a normal weight adult male indicates that he is composed of 60% water and only 15% fat. Optimal weight of fat in a normal weight female is 25%. In a typical obese male of 120 kg, fat accounts for 40% of the weight. Note the slight increases in protein and body water.

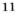 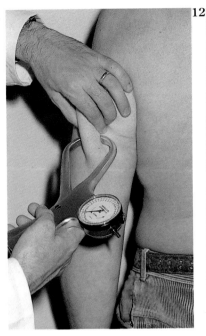 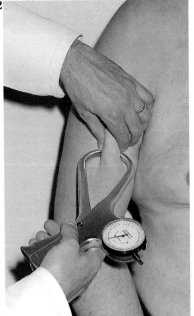 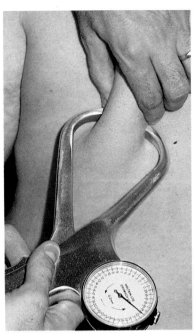

11 Skinfold thickness measured by Harpenden calipers can be used to measure body fat. The best established system is to measure the skinfold thickness of four sites. **Triceps skinfold** is measured half way between the acromial and olecranon processes. A fold of skin and subcutaneous tissue is pinched between the operator's thumb and forefinger. The grip is maintained with the left hand while the right hand relaxes the pressure of the calipers.

12 Biceps skinfold thickness is measured in the same place as the triceps skinfold but at the front of the arm with the hand supinated.

13 Subscapular skinfold thickness is measured at a 45° angle to the vertical at the lower angle of the left scapula.

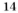 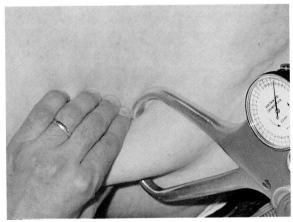

14 Suprailiac skinfold thickness is measured in the horizontal plane just above the iliac crest in the mid axillary line on the left side.

Table 5. Skinfold percentage fat

Skinfolds (mm)	Males (age in years)				Females (age in years)			
	17-29	30-39	40-49	50 +	16-29	30-39	40-49	50 +
15	4.8	—	—	—	10.5	—	—	—
20	8.1	12.2	12.2	12.6	14.1	17.0	19.8	21.4
25	10.5	14.2	15.0	15.6	16.8	19.4	22.2	24.0
30	12.9	16.2	17.7	18.6	19.5	21.8	24.5	26.6
35	14.7	17.7	19.6	20.8	21.5	23.7	26.4	28.5
40	16.4	19.2	21.4	22.9	23.4	25.5	28.2	30.3
45	17.7	20.4	23.0	24.7	25.0	26.9	29.6	31.9
50	19.0	21.5	24.6	26.5	26.5	28.2	31.0	33.4
55	20.1	22.5	25.9	27.9	27.8	29.4	32.1	34.6
60	21.2	23.5	27.1	29.2	29.1	30.6	33.2	35.7
65	22.2	24.3	28.2	30.4	30.2	31.6	34.1	36.7
70	23.1	25.1	29.3	31.6	31.2	32.5	35.0	37.7
75	24.0	25.9	30.3	32.7	32.2	33.4	35.9	38.7
80	24.8	26.6	31.2	33.8	33.1	34.3	36.7	39.6
85	25.5	27.2	32.1	34.8	34.0	35.1	37.5	40.4
90	26.2	27.8	33.0	35.8	34.8	35.8	38.3	41.2
95	26.9	28.4	33.7	36.6	35.6	36.5	39.0	41.9
100	27.6	29.0	34.4	37.4	36.4	37.2	39.7	42.6
105	28.2	29.6	35.1	38.2	37.1	37.9	40.4	43.3
110	28.8	30.1	35.8	39.0	37.8	38.6	41.0	43.9
115	29.4	30.6	36.4	39.7	38.4	39.1	41.5	44.5
120	30.0	31.1	37.0	40.4	39.0	39.6	42.0	45.1
125	30.5	31.5	37.6	41.1	39.6	40.1	42.5	45.7
130	31.0	31.9	38.2	41.8	40.2	40.6	43.0	46.2
135	31.5	32.3	38.7	42.4	40.8	41.1	43.5	46.7
140	32.0	32.7	39.2	43.0	41.3	41.6	44.0	47.2
145	32.5	33.1	39.7	43.6	41.8	42.1	44.5	47.7
150	32.9	33.5	40.2	44.1	42.3	42.6	45.0	48.2
155	33.3	33.9	40.7	44.6	42.8	43.1	45.4	48.7
160	33.7	34.3	41.2	45.1	43.3	43.6	45.8	49.2
165	34.1	34.6	41.6	45.6	43.7	44.0	46.2	49.6
170	34.5	34.8	42.0	46.1	44.1	44.4	46.6	50.0
175	34.9	—	—	—	—	44.8	47.0	50.4
180	35.3	—	—	—	—	45.2	47.4	50.8
185	35.6	—	—	—	—	45.6	47.8	51.2
190	35.9	—	—	—	—	45.9	48.2	51.6
195	—	—	—	—	—	46.2	48.5	52.0
200	—	—	—	—	—	46.5	48.8	52.4
205	—	—	—	—	—	—	49.1	52.7
210	—	—	—	—	—	—	49.4	53.0

Table 5 Skinfold percentage fat is calculated from the sum of the four skinfolds using the table published originally by Durnin and Wormersley (ref. 4).

15

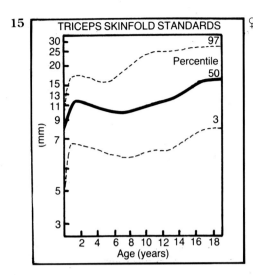
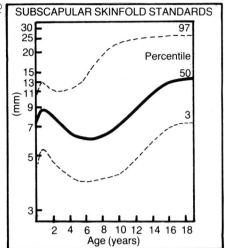

15 Skinfold thickness measurements for triceps and subscapular regions in **children** can be assessed on standard charts. Both measurements should be done since triceps alone is unreliable as there are ethnic differences in fat distribution in children between the trunk and limbs.

16

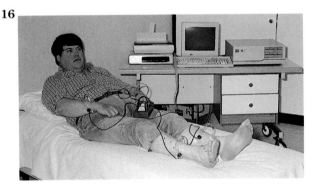

16 Impedance analysis is a simple, safe and relatively inexpensive method to measure body composition. This technique depends on the difference in electrical conductivity of lean tissue which is a good conductor, and fat which is a nonconductor. Electrodes are attached to hand and feet and a minute current is passed between the electrodes. The resistance is measured from the voltage drop.

17

BODY COMPOSITION			
	Sex: Male		
	Height: 5' 9''		
	Weight: 264 lbs		
	D.O.B.:		

Measurements

Physical (cm)		Conductivity	
Arm length	= 36.0		
Wrist girth	= 19.6	Upper body	= 29
Forearm Girth	= 31.5	Mid Body	= 35
Biceps Girth	= 39.3	Lower Body	= 34
Chest Girth	= 129		
Waist Girth	= 119	Fitness Tests	
Buttocks Girth	= 128		
Thigh Girth	= 59.8	Step Test	=
Calf Girth	= 44.8	Flexibility	=
Leg Length	= 94.0	Str-Lf Test	=
		Str-Rt Test	=

Goal Tabulations		Percentage Fat
% Fat	Body Fat (lbs to lose)	40.5%
		Lean Body Mass
40.5	0.0	157 lbs
38.5	8.6	
36.5	16.6	**Results**
34.5	24.2	Extra-cellular water = 41 lbs.
32.5	31.3	Intra-cellular water = 71 lbs.
30.5	38.0	Protein, muscle, etc = 34 lbs.
28.5	44.3	Other (bones, etc) = 11 lbs.
26.5	50.3	Total Fat = 107 lbs.
24.5	56.0	
22.5	61.3	
`marks your current position		

17 Output from BMR 2000 impedance analyser showing composition of an obese adult man.

18

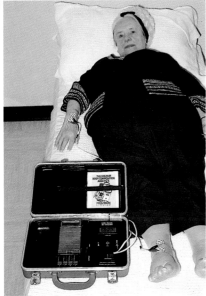

Table 6. Methods for measuring fat and lean tissue
Skinfold thickness
Impedance analysis
Water immersion plethysmograph
Total body composition
Neutron activation
Quatelet's index
Infrared interactance
Computer assisted tomography
Magnetic Nuclear Resonance

18 Impedance analysis measured by use of Holtain portable equipment. This machine gives a direct measurement of impedance which can then be used to calculate body composition using known equations for children and for adults.

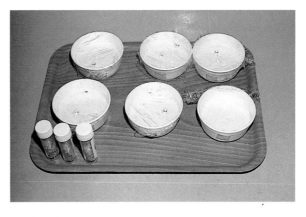

19 Intake can be accurately controlled by providing a liquid or semiliquid diet. This is feasible for a metabolic unit but unacceptable for use outside a closed environment as subjects find it too tedious and boring.

20

FOR EXAMPLE		
DAY OF THE WEEK	Sunday	
DATE		
TIME	AMOUNT	FOOD, DRINK
7.30 a.m.	1 rasher	back bacon fried
	2 slices	white toast, Mother's Pride, thin cut
	1tsp on each	butter spread thin
	2tsp on each	marmalade, Silver Shred
	1 teacupful	Kelloggs cornflakes
	1 cup	milk
10 a.m.	5tbs	beef stew with onions and carrots
	2tbs	cauliflower, fresh boiled
	3 pieces	potato boiled
	G (1½ inch deep)	home-made apple pie, crust top and bottom
	4tbs	custard
6.30 p.m.	½E by E (or 4x1x½ inch)	cheddar cheese
	10 slices (about 1 inch)	cucumber, peeled
	2 slices 1½ AxB thick	cold roast pork, fat eaten
	1pkt	Golden Wonder potato crisps (7p)
	1 slice ½G size	home-made Dundee cake
9 p.m.	2 squares	Cadbury's milk choc 14p bar
	¾pint	milk used all day

20 Intake is measured during a normal life style by having the subject weigh and record the food consumed. This is more accurate than the other method where a diet history is taken; this can underestimate intake by about one-third. The difficulty with weighing and recording is that it tends to inhibit food intake. Probably more reliable information about habitual energy intake can be derived from measurements of energy expenditure, taking into account changes in weight. (A to G refer to the actual size of the food portion.

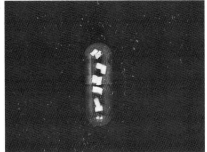

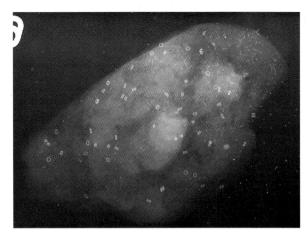

21 & 22 Faecal energy loss measurements show that these are normally about 5% of intake and that lean and obese subjects on similar diets absorb similar amounts. To collect stools accurately is best done by having the subject swallow capsules containing radio-opaque pellets (**21**), ther collecting and radiographing stools (**22**) until the number of pellets swallowed has been excreted.

Table 7. Calorimeter printed output

Time min	CO2 prod.	O2 cons.	R.Q.	H.P. kj/min
1	.255	.366	.697	7.224
2	.252	.373	.675	7.327
3	.222	.295	.751	5.894
4	.204	.267	.765	5.343
5	.226	.307	.735	6.115
6	.192	.248	.776	4.976
7	.188	.225	.834	4.534
8	.208	.258	.808	5.211
9	.188	.239	.788	4.815
10	.189	.248	.763	4.966
11	.182	.250	.730	4.963
12	.198	.265	.747	5.270
13	.188	.247	.760	4.942
14	.200	.256	.781	5.150
15	.194	.255	.758	5.110
16	.178	.236	.753	4.720
17	.176	.250	.704	4.940
18	.184	.259	.709	5.124
19	.178	.247	.722	4.898
20	.178	.261	.681	5.128
21	.193	.265	.730	5.260
22	.176	.248	.712	4.906
23	.195	.271	.721	5.376
24	.169	.247	.682	4.863
25	.165	.243	.677	4.772
26	.209	.271	.770	5.432

Table 7 Calorimeter printed output from the Ninewells machine shows oxygen consumed and carbon dioxide exhaled by the subject, respiratory quotient (RQ) and the calculated metabolic rate in Kj/min.

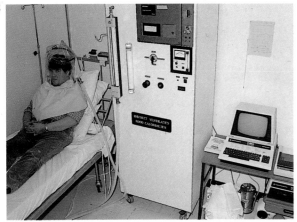

23 Ventilated hood indirect calorimeter. Air is pumped through the plastic hood worn by the subject. After the air is dried (vertical white column) it is sampled and analysed for oxygen by paramagnetic analysis and carbon dioxide by infra-red spectroscopy. Energy expenditure is computed automatically in this machine housed in the Department of Medicine, Ninewells Hospital, Dundee, so that minute by minute analysis is available.

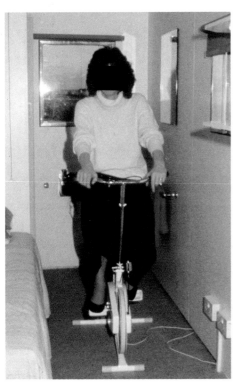

24 Direct calorimetery. The subject lives in an enclosed small chamber or room especially constructed so that heat output and gaseous exchange can be accurately measured and from this energy expenditure computed. Such a room allows the energy expenditure of various activities such as cycling, as shown, to be measured accurately.

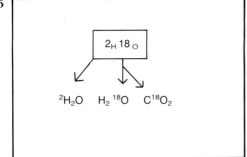

25 Doubly-labelled water technique is used to measure free living energy expenditure. The subject drinks a quantity of water in the form of deuterium and ^{18}oxygen, both heavy isotopes (hence $^{2}H\ ^{18}O$). The deuterium (^{2}H) is lost in water excretion in an exponential fashion (linear on log-linear paper). The ^{18}oxygen is lost not only in excreted water but also as expired carbon dioxide, hence more ^{18}oxygen is lost than deuterium. From the differences, the amount of carbon dioxide produced can be calculated and from this the energy expenditure measured.

2 Overview of Essential Obesity

Table 8 shows the numerous causes of obesity which will be discussed and illustrated in this and the following three chapters. Essential (idiopathic) obesity accounts for 99% of obese patients; so what is known about their obesity? In all obese individuals weight gain requires an energy intake in excess of energy expended over a prolonged period of time. Controversy arises over whether some individuals with a propensity for obesity have a lower energy expenditure at the outset and hence gain weight rapidly on an energy intake which others may find equal to their expenditure and hence show no weight gain whatsoever. Such a situation has been reported in some pre-obese individuals, both in infancy and in adulthood, and also in some normal weight individuals who have been previously obese (viz post obese).

Nevertheless, recent reports clearly indicate a degree of variability in energy expenditure in the

---

Table 8 Causes of Obesity

Essential (simple or idiopathic)
Multifactorial, inheritance, racial.

Genetic
Prader-Willi
Laurence-Moon Biedl
Alström
Morgagni-Stewart-Morel
DIDMOAD
Carpenter's Syndrome
Cohen's Syndrome

Mental Retardation
e.g. Down's
     Hurler's

Physical Disability
e.g. Spina bifida   Paraplegic

Hypothalamic
Trauma
Inflammation — meningitis
               encephalitis
               tuberculosis
               syphilis
Infiltration
             — sarcoidosis
               histiocytosis X
Tumours   — craniopharyngioma
               astrocytoma
Leukaemic leucodystrophy

Endocrine
Hypothalamus and pituitary — Growth hormone failure
                             Laron dwarf
                             Hypogonadotrophic
                               hypogonadism (Kallman)
                             Hyperprolactinaemia
                             Cushing's disease
                             Hypopituitarism
Thyroid   — Cretin
                             Primary and secondary
                               hypothyroidism
                             Rarely thyrotoxicosis

Endocrine cont.

Parathyroid   — Pseudohypoparathyroidism
                     Pseudo-pseudo
                       hypoparathyroidism
Adrenal   — Cushing's syndrome
Ovaries   — Polycystic ovarian syndrome
                     Postmenopausal
                     Turner's syndrome
Testes   — Primary hypogonadal
                     Klinefelter's syndrome
                     Sertoli cell only syndrome
                     Noonan's syndrome

Metabolic
Diabetes mellitus therapy
Nesidioblastoma
Insulinoma
Beckwith-Wiedemann syndrome
Hyperlipidaemia III and IV

Drugs
Sulphonylurea
Insulin
Oestrogen
Contraceptive pill
Alcohol
Corticosteroids
Cyproheptadine
Sodium valproate
Nonselective beta adrenergic blockade
Phenothiazines
Tricyclic antidepressants

Abnormal fat distribution
Multiple lipomatosis
Partial lipodystrophy

Painful fat
Dercum's disease

obese population some below and some above the average indicating that a reduction in energy expenditure certainly cannot explain the obesity of many individuals. If appetite varies as much as energy expenditure in an obese population then possibly this explains, in a simple manner, the diverse nature of the aetiology of obesity. Studies on twins indicate a degree of genetic involvement in the development of obesity but this is only one of possibly many factors involved in the development of so called 'idiopathic' obesity with environmental influences also playing a role.

Emphasis has been placed on an aetiological role of brown fat which is a potent thermogenic tissue in rodents. Obesity in certain strains of animals such as the ob/ob mouse is due to both hyperphagia and a major defect in the thermogenic activity of brown fat such that less of the food eaten is burnt off as heat. Certainly in adult man brown fat is present but is thought to contribute little to man's daily energy expenditure and many do not consider that by itself it could account for the variations in energy expenditure reported. Active research is underway to try and find ways of increasing thermogenesis in man as an effective method of increasing energy expenditure enhancing weight loss while on a diet.

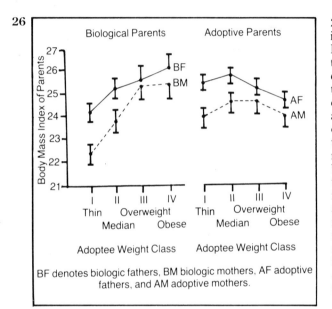

26

BF denotes biologic fathers, BM biologic mothers, AF adoptive fathers, and AM adoptive mothers.

26 Genetic and family environmental influences investigated by Stunkard and his colleagues in 540 adult Danish adoptees where information was available on both the biological and the adopted parents. The adoptees were divided into four groups depending on whether they were thin, average, overweight or obese, each group being then compared with the body mass index of the biological and adoptive parents. Note the close association of the weight of the adoptees with their biological parents, the heavier the parents, the heavier the adoptee. For biological mothers the association was highly significant ($p < 0.0001$) but less so for biological fathers ($p < 0.02$). In contrast, there was no apparent relation between the body mass index of the adoptive parents and the weight of the adoptees. The conclusion was that genetic influences are important in determining body fatness and that childhood family environment alone has little effect in this Danish society where food was in abundance. The latter is important since environmental factors do influence genetic expression where food availability may alter dependency on the family's attitude, finances and education (ref. 5).

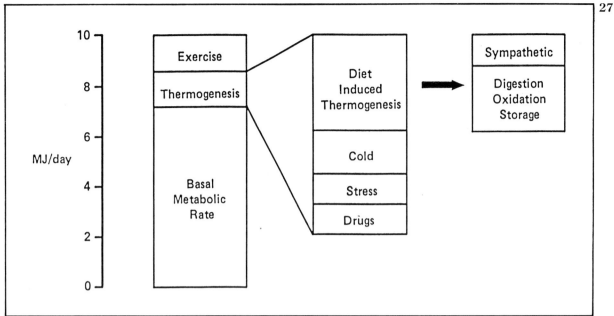

27 The major component of energy expenditure is the basal metabolic rate accounting for about 70% of the 24 hr energy output. This basal metabolism reflects the energy cost of synthetic activities such as protein synthesis, mechanical work (e.g. cardiac action) and sodium pumping across cells, which are all activities necessary to keep the body alive. A variable amount of expenditure somewhere in the region of 10% is the result of exercise.

The other 20% is the result of thermogenic activities such as diet induced thermogenesis (i.e. the heat released when food is digested, oxidised and stored) and the heat produced in response to cold, stressful situations and drugs (e.g. smoking and caffeine). As the sympathetic system plays a major role in the thermogenic component of energy expenditure scientists often use infused catecholamines to measure its significance.

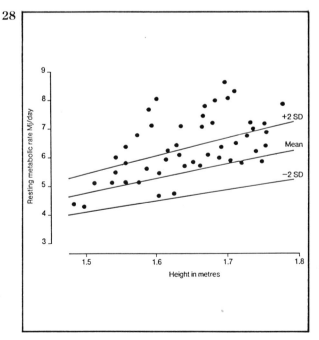

28 The **basal metabolic rate** is closely related to the size of the **lean body mass** which comprises muscle and other proteinaceous structures. As obese individuals often have an increased lean mass (see **Table 4**) their whole body basal metabolic rate is elevated. In this figure the basal metabolic rate of obese subjects is shown in comparison to the mean and ± 2 SD of normal weight individuals. None of the obese had a subnormal metabolic rate and in over one-third the metabolic rate was markedly elevated. This would suggest that 24 hr energy expenditure is elevated in many obese individuals (ref. 6).

	Intake	24 hr Energy Expenditure	Basal Metabolic Rate	Activity and Thermo-genic Maintenance
Lean (13)	7.85	7.99	5.65	2.26
Obese (9)	6.73	10.22	6.71	3.45

Table 9. Intake (MJ/24 hr) compared with expenditure (MJ/24 hr) in lean and obese

Whether the **obese eat more than lean** has been examined by many but the study by Prentice and his colleagues (**Table 9**) was novel in also measuring free living total energy expenditure by the doubly labelled water ($^2H_2$ ^{18}O) method. Intake was also assessed using the usual method of weighing all foods and fluids over a seven day period of study. The energy expenditure in the obese was 28% higher on average than the lean with higher resting metabolic rates, activity and maintenance expenditures. Yet energy intake was 34% lower than expenditure in the obese and actually less than in the lean as others have previously reported. If the intake measured in the obese was a true reflection of their average intake then the obese should

have rapidly lost weight which was not the case. The lean group's intake closely parallelled their energy expenditure so the technique used to measure intake appeared fairly accurate. Hence, the obese must have under reported their intake, a finding now reported by others who estimate that the obese eat on average 20% more than lean people. This experiment has been supported by others using direct calorimetry where the obese have been shown to have higher energy expenditures than the lean. However, this does not exclude some degree of variability in the obese, nor does it exclude some thermic abnormality in the pre-obese stage which might also be unmasked in the post-obese state (ref. 7).

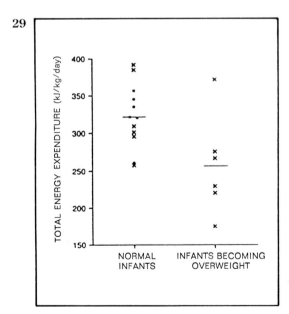

29

29 Pre-obese infant energy expenditure at three months of age was studied by Roberts and her colleagues using the doubly labelled water method. The subjects were infants of 6 lean (■) and 12 overweight (x) mothers, recruited into their study soon after birth. They studied the infants up to one year of age, dividing them at this age into two groups depending on whether they became overweight or not. They then compared each with the total energy expenditure measured at three months of age before any of the infants became fat. They noted that those who became fat at one year of age were born to overweight mothers and that energy expenditure at three months of age was on average 20.7% lower in those infants who became overweight (p < 0.05) at one year. They suggest from this data that reduced energy expenditure may be an important factor in the rapid weight gain during the first year of life of infants born to overweight mothers. Note the variability in energy expenditure in both groups of infants, clearly indicating that a reduced energy expenditure is not the whole story (ref. 9).

Table 10. Thermic Response in Normal Weight Adult Subjects			
	Percent increase above resting metabolic rate		
	Intake (MJ/day)	Meal (2 MJ)	Ephedrine (0.25 mg/kg)
High energy intake	15.0	21.6	15.7
Low energy intake	6.9	8.2	5.2
		$p < 0.025$	$p < 0.05$

Table 10 Energetically efficient individuals have been reported. Morgan and her colleagues studied 16 adult, male, postgraduate students and staff at Southampton University, UK, selected on their level of food intake. Half were lean and habitually consumed large amounts of food whereas the others, though lean, admitted to a weight problem and regularly consumed a lower than average food intake. They used indirect calorimetry to measure each subject's response to a 2 MJ meal and to ephedrine administration. Note the reduced thermic response to both a meal and ephedrine in the low energy intake group, suggesting that these individuals were energetically more efficient (ref. 8).

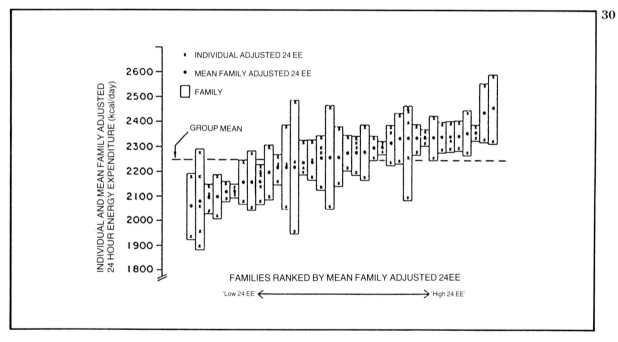

30 The heterogeneity of man is reflected in the wide variation of energy expenditure seen. This has been most effectively shown by Ravussen and colleagues who studied 24 hr energy expenditure by direct calorimetry in 94 individuals from 36 families of Southwestern American Indians, a population prone to obesity. Note the wide variation in energy expenditure between families in this population. About one-third of families had an energy expenditure below the average whereas others had energy expenditure significantly above the population's mean. If followed up for two years then energy expenditure was found to predict the rate of change in body weight ($r = -0.39$, $p < 0.001$). For instance, if a person had a 24 hr energy expenditure 200 kcal (0.8 MJ) below the average, that person had a four-fold increased risk of gaining more than 7.5 kg than another whose expenditure was 200 kcal (0.8 MJ) above the average. They also found that energy expenditure aggregated in families suggesting a definite familial predisposition (ref. 11).

Table 11. Whole body calorimetry and intake in post-obese (MJ/24 hr)				
	Energy Intake	**Energy Expenditure**		
		Sedentary	Normal	Normal & aerobics
Lean (16)	8.0	6.4	7.8	8.8
Post-obese (16)	5.4	5.3	6.6	7.5
		↓ 17%	↓ 15%	↓ 15%

Table 11 Energy expenditure and intake in the post-obese was recently investigated in depth by Geissler, Miller and Shah. They studied 16 lean and 16 post-obese women each of similar weight (61.8 vs 60.8 kg); body mass index 22.4 vs 22.5) and lean body mass (45.6 vs 43.5 kg respectively). Energy expenditure was measured in a room respirometer, a type of direct calorimeter, during three different levels of activity. Intake was measured by weighed food inventory over a 7 day period. The post-obese had lower energy expenditures at all three levels of activity than the matched lean group and their energy intake balanced energy output in the sedentary state. The conlusion was that the post-obese had to eat less to maintain their new reduced weight. This study suggests that there are some individuals with a propensity for obesity who do have a more efficient energy system and to remain at a normal weight must eat less than others (ref. 10).

Conclusion

There is such heterogeneity in the pool of obese individuals that it is most unlikely that a thermic abnormality reducing energy expenditure, will be found in all, some having hyperphagia to a greater degree than others to account for their obesity. The balance between metabolic efficiency and appetite will determine whether obesity develops or not. The situation in man is quite unlike that in animal research where pure bred rodents are used which have a distinct genetic tendency for obesity and therefore all show the same specific defect.

31

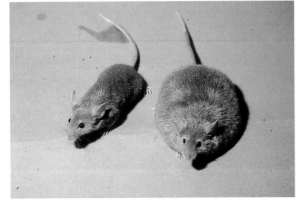

31 The ob/ob mouse is one of many laboratory bred strains with a distinct genetic obesity trait. The ob (obese) gene is inherited as a recessive condition. One offspring in four of a heterozygous mating is homozygous for the ob gene (i.e. ob/ob) and subsequently develops gross obesity. This picture illustrates the ob/ob mouse with its lean sibling.

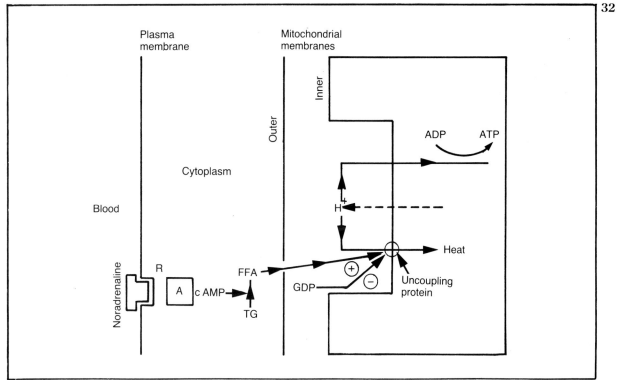

32 The brown fat proton shunt is set at a reduced rate in the ob/ob mouse and this limits the rodent's capacity for non-shivering thermogenesis hence promoting obesity. In the brown fat cell noradrenaline acts on a receptor (R) to activate adenyl cyclase (A) which in turn stimulates lipolysis. The released fatty acids activate a unique proton shunt in the inner mitochondrial membrane which allows protons (H^+) to re-enter the mitochondrial matrix releasing energy as heat. GDP, a purine nucleotide, inhibits this uncoupling protein (UP).

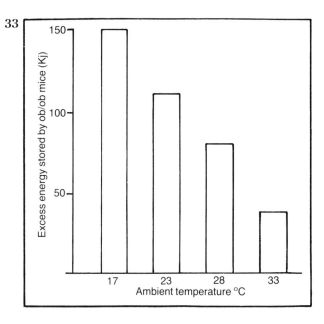

33 Defective thermogenic capacity increases energy storage as illustrated by Thurlby and Trayhurn. Groups of lean and ob/ob mice were pairfed for 10 days while housed at different environmental temperatures. At thermoneutrality (33°C) the excess energy stored by the ob/ob mutants is slight (41 kj). As the ambient temperature decreases, the thermic activity of brown fat increases to keep the animals warm. As the ob/ob mutant has a defect in this capacity it has less in reserve to burn off excess food as heat and therefore the obese mice store progressively more energy in comparison to their lean littermates as the ambient temperature is reduced. At 4°C the ob/ob mice just cannot cope and will rapidly die from hypothermia (ref. 13).

Table 12.	GDP binding (pmol/mg mitochondrial protein)					
Mice			**Rats**			
		Normal diet		Overfed		
Lean	ob/ob	Warm	Cold	Warm	Cold	
107	50	53	250	135	238	

Table 12 GDP binding was studied by Brooks and colleagues as a measure of brown fat proton shunt capacity. If rats are overfed then GDP binding rises, as it also does if rats are exposed to cold (4°C). In the ob/ob mouse GDP binding is low, over 50% less than in lean littermates kept in a warm (24°C) environment clearly indicating a thermogenic defect in brown fat in the ob/ob strain (ref. 12).

34

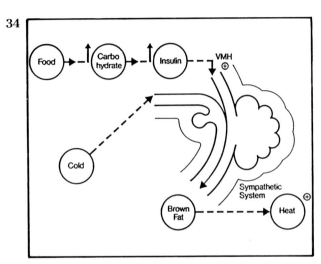

34 Hypothalamic role. In rodents, excess carbohydrate increases insulin, which stimulates the sympathetic system by acting on insulin-sensitive neurones in the ventromedial hypothalamic area (the classical 'satiety' area). The increased sympathetic activity stimulates brown fat heat production. Cold exposure acts via the temperature sensitive area of the hypothalamus to stimulate the sympathetic system which then activates heat production from brown fat. Hence rats made diabetic with streptozotocin have a reduced thermogenic drive to overfeeding which is corrected by giving insulin.

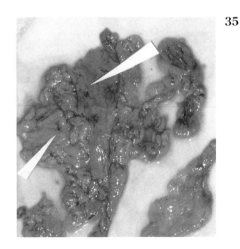

35

35 Human brown fat, which is plentiful in human babies, appears to diminish with age but can still be detected in adult man, especially in the perinephric fat deposits. In this picture the brown colour of the fat is visible amongst white fat.

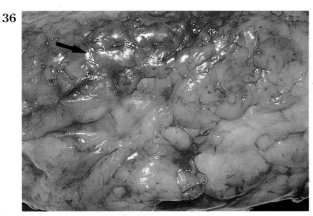

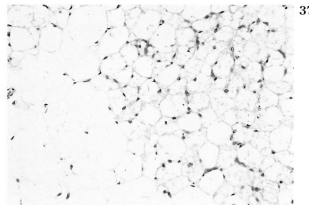

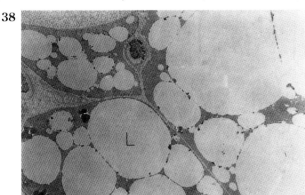

36 Brown fat in adult man tends to be found interspersed histologically amongst white fat cells, although large clumps of brown fat can often be seen with the naked eye. This is a kidney surrounded by perinephric fat showing a large clump of brown fat (arrow).

37 Human perinephric adipose tissue stained with haematocyclin and eosin showing white fat on the left and brown fat to the right. Note the multilocular lipid deposits and the more abundant cytoplasm of the brown fat tissue (× 450).

38 Electron micrograph of human perirenal brown fat showing multilocular lipid droplets (L) (× 3000).

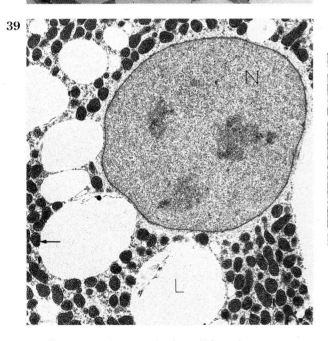

39 Electron micrograph of a cell from human perirenal brown adipose tissue showing the nucleus (N), numerous dense mitochondria (arrowed) and multiocular lipid droplets (L). Note the orderly shelflike disposition of mitochondrial cristae (× 3100).

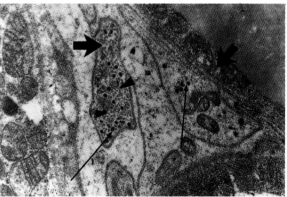

40 Electron micrograph of Schwann axon bundle in an intercellular space between brown adipocytes. The bundle contains axons (heavy arrows) exhibiting terminal features, namely large diameter (800-1000 A), dense cored vesicles (long arrows) and small diameter (400-600 Å), clear vesicles (arrowheads). Peripheral cytoplasm of brown adipocytes (BF) surrounds the axon bundle (× 26000) (ref. 14).

41

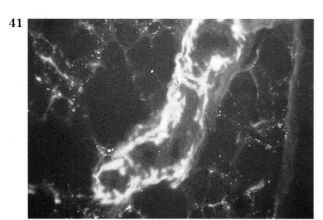

41 Catecholaminergic nervous input into adult human perirenal brown fat as shown by the blue fluorescence in the micrograph of sucrose potassium glycoxylic acid-treated tissue. Note the dense plexus surrounding the artery and in the periphery beaded, fluorescent fibres are also seen between individual adipocytes. The brown autofluorescent bodies are lipofuscin particles within adipocytes. Possibly these bodies along with the dense mitochondria produce the brown colour of so-called 'brown fat' (× 750) (ref. 14 for details).

42

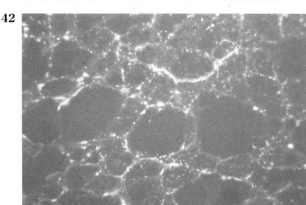

42 Brown fat in a patient with phaeochromocytoma. The brown fat, which was found interposed between islands of white adipose tissue, was conspicuous by virtue of the prolific catecholaminergic innervation, shown up as beaded blue fluorescence in contrast to the sparsely innervated white fat (× 750) (ref. 15, 16).

43 & 44 Neuropeptide Y is found in human, brown adipose tissue. A haemotoxylin and eosin preparation (**43**) shows the area studied, namely a section of brown fat with major arterial supply. Fluorescent-prepared slide using antisera against neuropeptide Y shows up this peptide's distribution as a yellow fluoresence (**44**). Note the prominent periarterial as well as the beaded parenchymal distribution between individual brown adipocytes. Nerves containing neuropeptide Y follow a similar distribution to catecholaminergic fibres. Both neuropeptide Y and catecholaminergic nerves control the blood supply to brown fat (× 750) (ref. 16).

43

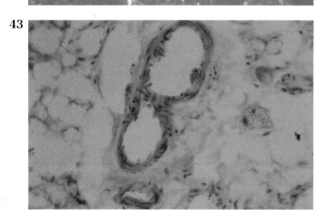

45 Calcitonin gene related peptide (CGRP) has also been found in human, brown adipose tissue. CGRP immunoreactivity is seen as a yellow, fluorescent, fine-beaded plexus on the walls of the supply artery to this section of brown fat (× 750). Bombesin has also been found in human brown adipose tissue (ref. 16).

44

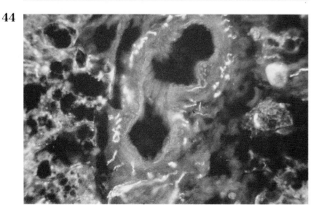

45

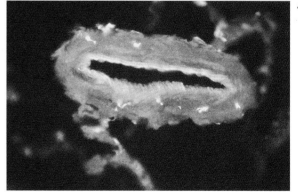

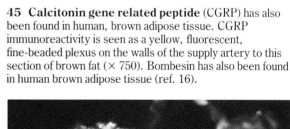

46

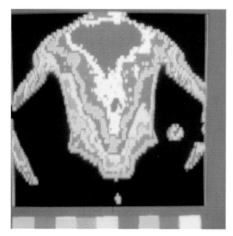

46 Thermocamera can detect heat generated over the upper back after the ingestion of ephedrine. Note the hotter area (red and white) over the interscapular area. A more precise method, which circumvents vasomotor skin changes, is to insert fine needle thermocouples deep into the interscapular tissue.

Table 13. GDP Binding (nmol/GDP/mg mitochondrial protein)		
Adult	**Guinea Pigs**	
Humans	*Warm*	*Cold*
0.13 - 0.30	0.10	0.75

Table 13 GDP Binding is a measure of the activity of the uncoupling protein specific to brown fat and necessary for its potent thermogenic activity. In adult man GDP binding ranges from 0.13 to 0.30 nmol/mg protein which, when compared with the values found in warm and cold adapted guinea pigs, suggests that man is in a warm adapted state with only slight brown fat thermogenic activity (ref. 17).

47

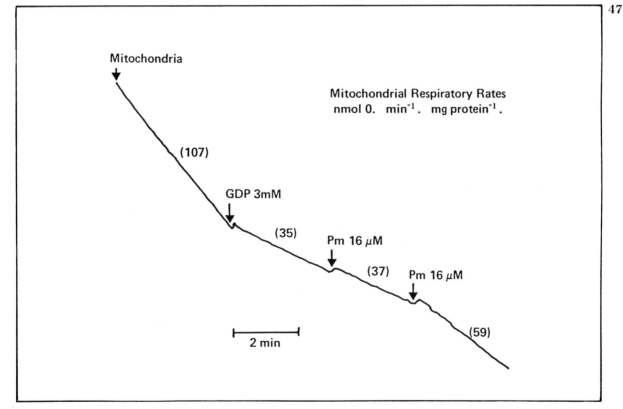

47 Actual **tracing of the respiratory rate of human brown fat mitochondria.** This is measured using a tetra phenylphosphonium sensitive electrode and the proton current generated by the respiratory chain is measured with an oxygen electrode. The figure in brackets represents the respiratory activity in nmol O./min/mg mitochondrial proton. Note the partial inhibition of respiratory activity by GDP and its reactivation by two additions of palmitic acid (PM) (ref. 17).

Table 14. Estimated contribution to in vivo respiration of human perinephric fat.

Perinephric fat used 22-212 (mean 72) $\mu l\, O_2^{-1}\, min^{-1}$		
	$ml\, O_2^{-1}\, min^{-1}$	Contributes
Resting metabolic rate	173-219	$< 0.04\%$
Noradrenaline infusion	14-49	$< 0.5\%$

Table 14 The thermogenic contribution of human brown fat is difficult to estimate precisely since one does not as yet know how much brown fat exists in adult man. In one experiment, measuring cytochrome C oxidase activity of human brown fat mitochondria from human perinephric fat depots, it was concluded that brown fat in adult man has very little thermogenic potential. This accounts for $<0.04\%$ of the oxygen utilised in the resting metabolic rate and less than $<0.5\%$ of the rise in oxygen utilised when noradrenaline (0.1 ug $min^{-1}\, kg^{-1}$ ideal weight) was infused. This suggests that brown fat in man is not that active but could be stimulated by suitable drugs if one compares man's level of activity with that of rabbits or guinea pigs (ref. 17).

Fat cell size, number and distribution

The observation that fat cell size and number could be altered by feeding patterns in neonatal rats led to the concept of hyperplastic and hypertrophic obesity. It was proposed that the development of obesity in infancy and early childhood was associated with an increased number of white adipocytes (hyperplastic obesity). As there were more fat cells, and since each retained a minimum of triglyceride, the result would be life-long obesity which was difficult, if not impossible, to treat effectively. This led to the erroneous idea that all fat babies become fat adults. Although obese children are at risk of becoming obese adults, this is not inevitable as epidemiological research has shown. Further studies also failed to confirm that moderately obese adults, who date the origin of their obesity to childhood, have a hypercellular adipocyte mass, although this is a feature of those with excessive obesity.

The second type of obesity, the adult onset type, was thought to be due to enlarged white adipocytes and not due to an increased number of cells (hypertrophic obesity). Research has shown that as the individual increases in weight there is an initial increase in fat cell size with existing adipocytes accommodating the accumulated fat until the individual's body weight has about doubled. With a further increase in weight fat cell numbers must increase to accommodate the fat. Thus, extremely obese subjects would be expected to show a hypercellular adipocyte picture whereas the moderately obese would show a hypertrophic situation.

Another difficulty was that fat cell size can vary considerably from one site to another with as much as 30% of patients having a two-fold difference in fat cell size between sites. Hence, a hyperplastic picture may be seen at one site and a hypertrophic picture at another. Overall this concept has little clinical consequence.

There is evidence to suggest that thigh fat in females plays an important role in providing lipids during pregnancy and lactation. The fat cells tend to be smaller in the thigh area and are less responsive to adrenaline induced lipolysis outside pregnancy and lactation. Such differences are also seen between subcutaneous and omental fat. Adipocytes from subcutaneous fat of the abdominal wall are more resistant to adrenaline induced lipolysis and more sensitive to insulin mediated antilipolysis than fat cells obtained ·simultaneously from the omentum. These findings may relate to the observation that obesity due to intra-abdominal fat deposition within the peritoneal cavity imposes a greater risk of hyperinsulinaemia, glucose intolerance, hypertriglyceridaemia and hypertension than does an equivalent amount of fat in the subcutaneous fat of the abdominal wall.

48

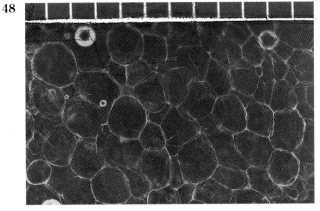

49

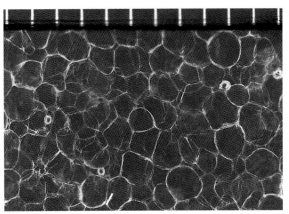

50

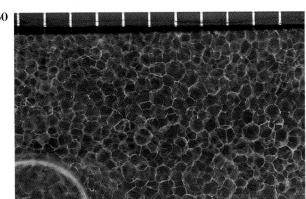

48 Percutaneous needle biopsy sample of subcutaneous, gluteal white fat shows the typical picture of 'hypertrophic' obesity. Large, white fat cells are seen. (Each scale division represents 100 μ.)

49 & 50 Percutaneous needle biopsy samples of fat are from the same patient taken simultaneously at hysterectomy operation. **49** was taken from subcutaneous fat of the abdominal wall whereas **50** was from omental fat. Note the small size of the omental adipocytes, a feature often seen. (Each scale division represents 100 μ.)

51

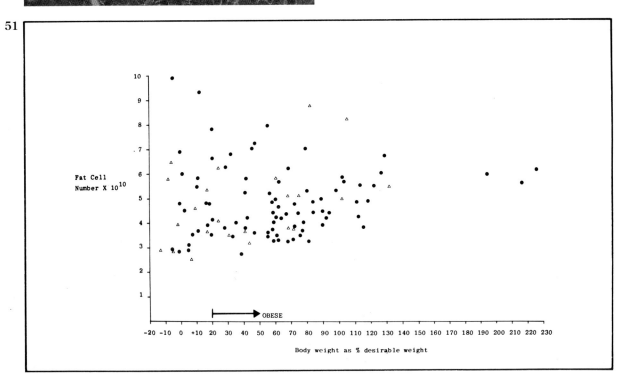

51 Total number of fat cells derived from the biopsy of four subcutaneous sites related to body weight; ● represents women, △ represents men. Note the wide scatter of fat cell numbers even in the non-obese. There was no suggestion that adults with childhood onset obesity had more cells than adults with adult onset type obesity (ref. 18).

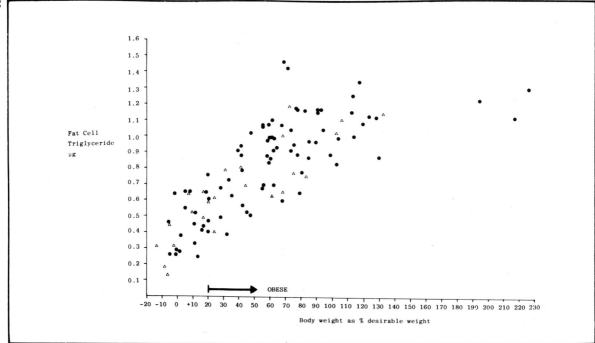

52 Total fat cell triglyceride as a measure of fat cell size related to body weight. As body weight increases there is progressive rise in lipid content of adipocytes till a plateau of an average 1.1 µg lipid is reached. After that plateau, fat cell number has to increase if extra fat is to be stored (ref. 18).

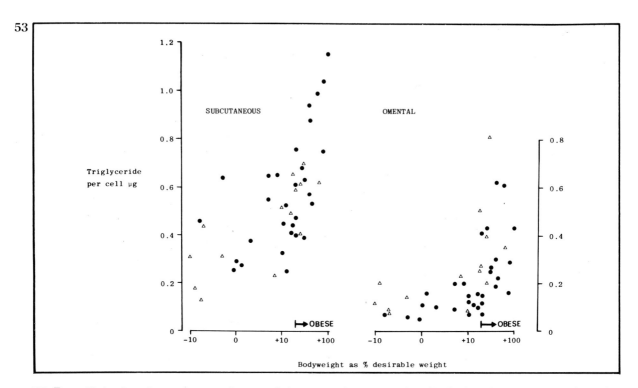

53 Fat cell size in subcutaneous and omental sites. Note that as obesity increases the fat cells in the subcutaneous sites fill with fat before the omental site (ref. 18).

Body shape

After puberty the fat distribution of males and females shows marked differences. Women store fat around the breast, hip and thigh regions until the menopause when abdominal obesity becomes more prevalent.

Nevertheless, some men can exhibit gynaecoid fat distribution and some women a central or android fat distribution.

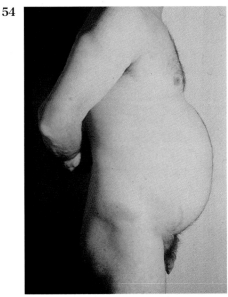

54 Abdominal fat distribution of a typical obese man produces a characteristic 'pot belly'.

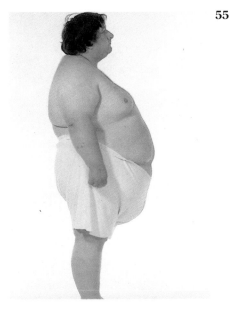

55 Massive male obesity is still associated with a central distribution of fat.

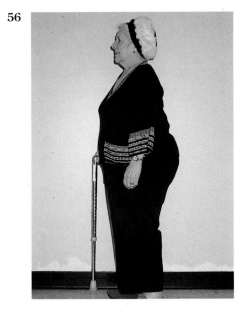

56 Gynaecoid fat distribution in this obese woman is sometimes referred to as 'peripheral' or '*pear*' obesity. The excess fat is mainly distributed around the hips, thighs and buttocks. See **18** for a frontal view of the same subject.

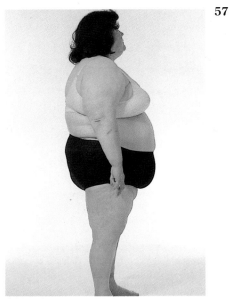

57 'Apple' or android obesity in a woman consists of a central or abdominal distribution of fat.

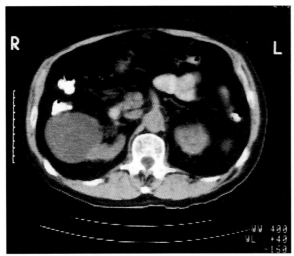

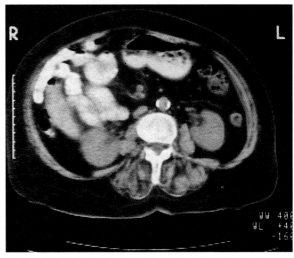

58 Computer assisted tomography (CAT) of a typical obese male patient shows that much fat is contained within the abdomen.

59 CAT of a typical obese female shows that fat is mainly subcutaneous with little intra-abdominal fat.

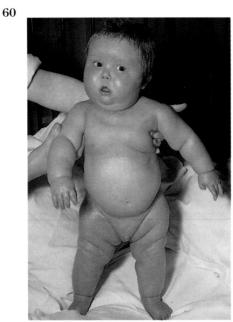

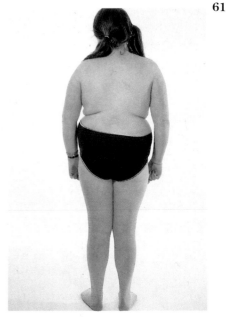

60 Fat babies do not necessarily become fat adults, although there is a definite risk of becoming overweight in later life. One study shows that 64% of overweight infants did not become fat adults but the other 36% did. This compared unfavourably with the incidence of 14% in those of average and light weight in infancy (ref. 19).

61 Adolescent obesity can be a problem, especially in girls. Unless diet is restricted and sound nutritional habits taught then such 'puppy fat' is unlikely to be carried through life, more so in girls than boys. Ten per cent of children are obese even if their parents are both of normal weight. The prevalence rate of obesity in childhood rises to 50% if one parent is obese and to 80% if both parents are obese.

3 Genetic Causes

Table 15. Genetic Causes of Obesity
Primary
Prader-Willi
Laurence-Moon-Biedl
Alström
DIDMOAD
Cohen
Carpenter
Morgagni-Stewart-Morel
Morel
Morgagni
Secondary
Mental retardation
Physical disability

Table 16. Some Features of Prader-Willi Syndrome

Cardinal	—	Hypotonia, obesity, hypogonadism, short stature, mental retardation
Gestation	—	Diminished intra-uterine movement Breech delivery Non-term delivery
Neonatal	—	Hypotonia Feeding problems Weak or absent cry
Facies	—	Narrow bifrontal diameter Strabismus Almond-shaped eyes Fish-shaped, open mouth
Body	—	Thick thighs Central obesity Small hands and feet Pin prick sensation reduced over arms and legs
Skeletal	—	Kyphoscoliosis Enamel hypoplasia and dental caries Short stature
CNS	—	Epilepsy Personality problems Mental retardation of variable degree Thermoregulation abnormalities
Endocrine	—	Diabetic glucose tolerance test Clinical diabetes Hypogonadism Testicular abnormalities
Chromosomes	—	Abnormalities on chromosome 15

Prader-Willi syndrome

This syndrome is characterised by neonatal hypotonia, hypogonadism, mental retardation, obesity and, in most, short stature. **Table 16** lists the major features that have been reported in this syndrome.

The disorder makes its appearance in infancy with feeding problems, hypotonia, diminished spontaneous movements and weak or absent cry. A higher than expected predominance of breech delivery has been reported (40%). Other associated features are diminished intra-uterine movements and non-term delivery. Motor development can be delayed with often delayed walking (two to four years of age). When the child becomes active enough to forage for food the major clinical problem, obesity and its consequences, become manifest. All cases are excessively fat and some to a gross degree. Most have an insatiable appetite so that food has to be locked away. There are reports of such patients eating from the dog's bowl and even from kitchen garbage destined as pigs' swill.

Most, but not all, are short, often below the 3rd centile on the height for age chart. Variants of Prader-Willi can present with normal height and variable mental retardation. The facies are characteristic with close-set, almond-shaped eyes, narrow bifrontal diameter, prominent nasal bridge, open, fish-shaped mouth and 40% are said to have stabismus.

Hands and feet are small in 80% (acromicra). The hands show a straight ulnar border compared with the normal slight curve. All patients have large thighs with the lower legs tapering to small feet. Pin prick sensation can be diminished in the arms and legs and this can result in sores over these areas, often secondarily infected from scratching. The skin texture is that of a hypogonadal person and is of a silky texture.

Scoliosis has been reported in up to 60% of cases. In some it is recognisable in early childhood but becomes most obvious in the adults affected. Enamel hypoplasia and dental caries have been reported.

The muscular hypotonia, which probably accounts for the reduced intra-uterine activity reported, has been investigated without any clear single abnormality found. Electron microscopical appearance of muscle biopsies has shown some abnormalities including sarcolemmal aggregates of mitochondria, tortuous irregular Z lines which can be found obliquely across the myofilaments, and limited areas of myofilament disorganisation. No excess glycogen has been reported.

Mental retardation is a universal finding and some 16% have epileptic fits. The children have a somewhat naive friendliness which continues into adult life, although some show episodes of sudden bursts of temper described as rages. Violence appears to be rare and none seems to be able to move quickly enough to injure other people. Intelligence testing places most in the lower range of normal in early childhood, but by the age of seven to eleven years most attend educationally subnormal or special schools.

Somnolence appears to be an almost universal accompaniment of the syndrome and often this can be the only respite from eating. Such somnolence is a problem especially in those who are grossly obese. Many die from cardiorespiratory failure secondary to their obesity and scoliosis. Possibly as many as 30% have a diabetic gluocse tolerance curve with about 10% being clinically diabetic.

The hypogonadism is often associated with cryptorchidism and appears to be due to some malfunction at the hypothalamic level with deficiency of LH and FSH (hypogonadotrophic hypogonadism). Nevertheless, there have been reports of normal and even elevated levels of LH and FSH, suggesting a primary gonadal abnormality may coexist. Some female patients have been reported to menstruate occasionally or even regularly and premature adrenarche and sexual precocity have also been recorded. Testicular biopsy has shown abnormalities such as interstitial cell defects, tubular atrophy, absence of the germinal cell layer and lack of spermatogenesis. Impaired thermoregulation in the cold has been reported, consistent possibly with some hypothalamic damage, although no structural lesion has been reported at necropsy. Prader-Willi syndrome is known to be familial. Twins, siblings, cousins have been reported, although rarely. Recently, abnormalities of chromosome 15 have been reported and many now consider the cause of the syndrome to be deletions in the 15th chromosome.

Treatment of this condition is difficult. The charm, apparent lack of appetite control and mental retardation of those affected make it very difficult to maintain any form of diet. Many cause havoc at home not only because food stores and garbage must be locked away but also because parents and siblings find their own plates raided. Appetite suppressants appear to be useless. Surgery can be successful although the complications are especially hazardous (ref. 20, 21).

62

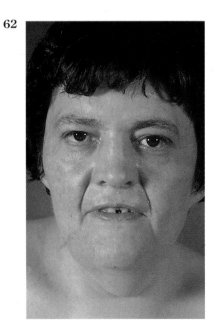

62 Prader-Willi syndrome. This 38 year old male patient shows the typical facial features of almond eyes, fish-shaped mouth and prominent nasal bridge. He also had marked dental caries. **62** to **68** are of same patient (ref. 21).

63

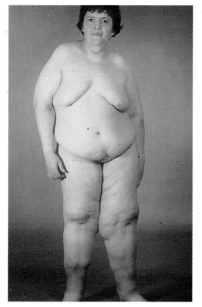

64

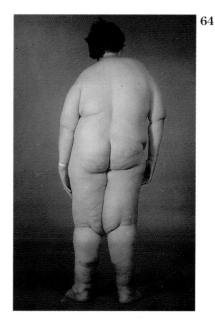

63 Prader-Willi. Standing showing gross obesity and fatty gynaecomastia (height 1.56 m, weight 104 kg). There is brawny oedema of the legs. Retardation in this patient was in the borderline area of subnormality (Weschler Adult Intelligence Scale IQ 77).

64 Prader-Willi. Rear view showing overall distribution of fat, especially notable on the thighs. There is also severe kyphoscoliosis.

65

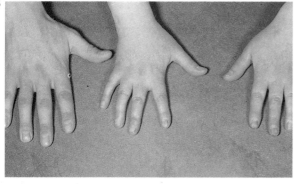

66

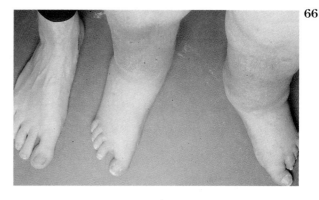

65 Prader-Willi. Diminutive hands compared to a normal adult.

66 Prader-Willi. Feet are also smaller than a normal adult as seen here. Note the tapering at the ankle region.

67 Prader-Willi. Secondary sexual development is poor. Voice is unbroken, no need to shave and testes not palpable. Phallus is small.

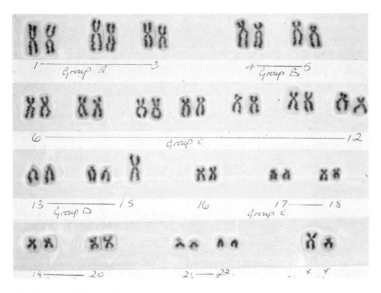

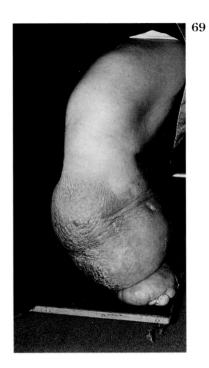

68 Prader-Willi. Karyotype is 45 XY (15q 15q) in the above patient. There is a large, metacentric chromosome due to translocation and centric fusion between the members of pair No. 15. Karyotype of the mother and father of this patient was normal (ref. 21).

69 Prader-Willi. Lymphoedema can be a problem as in this patient.

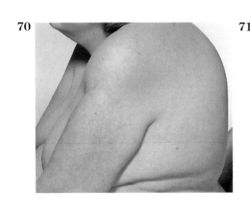

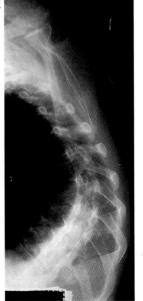

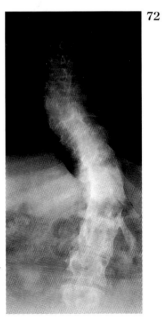

70 Prader-Willi. Marked kyphoscoliosis in this female patient led to respiratory problems. **71** and **72** are of this patient.

71 Prader-Willi. Lateral radiograph of kyphosis.

72 Prader-Willi. Radiograph showing severe degree of scoliosis.

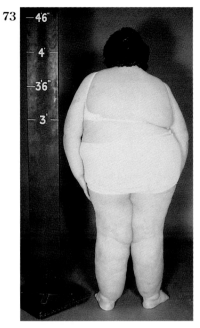

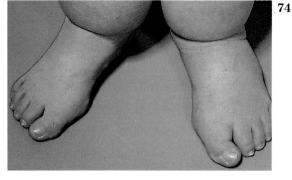

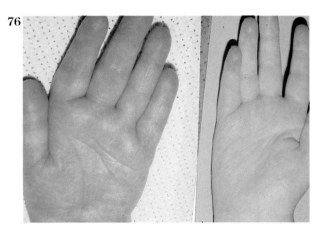

73 Prader-Willi. Adult female of marked short stature. Note the degree and distribution of the obesity and associated kyphoscoliosis.

74 Prader-Willi. Note again the tapering at the ankle and small feet in this female patient.

75 Prader-Willi. Early development of obesity in this child with central and thigh distribution.

76 Prader-Willi. The hands show a straight ulnar border compared with the normal subject curve. The hands are from two separate patients with this syndrome.

Laurence-Moon-Biedl syndrome

This syndrome can present with variable manifestations but is generally characterised by hypogonadism, retarded growth, obesity, mental retardation, polydactyly or syndactyly and visual impairment.

Total visual impairment can be delayed (mean age 30 years) and is due to retinal degeneration and retinitis pigmentosa. The extra endocrine features of this syndrome have been described in women with normal ovarian function and fertility and in males with normal testicular function and morphology. In those with hypogonadism the cause can be variable. In many there is a testicular lesion, whereas in others, features of hypogonadotrophic hypogonadism are apparent.

The aetiology of this syndrome is unknown although some aberration in chromosome number or morphology has been suggested since Laurence-Moon-Biedl and Turner's syndrome have occurred in one sibship. Nevertheless, recessive autosomal inheritance with incomplete penetrance has also been suggested.

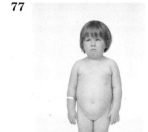

77

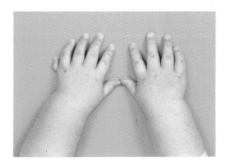

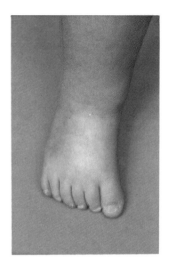

77 Laurence-Moon-Biedl syndrome. Showing obesity, genu valgum and polydactylism (supplementary little finger of left hand and six toes on the foot).

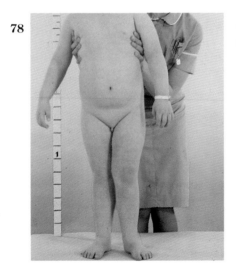

78

78 Laurence-Moon-Biedl. An older child showing the typical abdominal fat distribution.

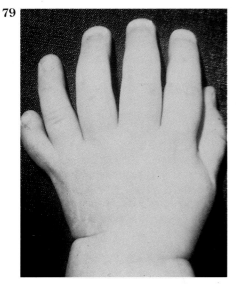

79 Polydactylism. The hands are small and exhibit a supplementary little finger on the left hand.

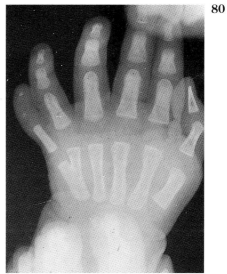
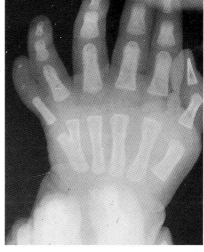

80 Radiograph of polydactylism in 79.

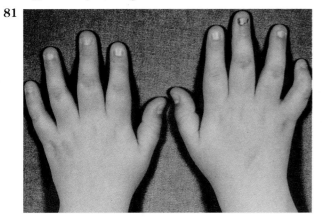

81 Laurence-Moon-Biedl. Variant with no polydactylism but curved fifth finger.

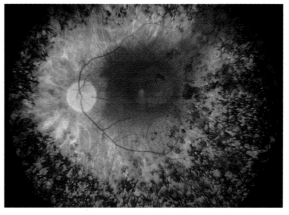

82 Retinitis Pigmentosa. Visual impairment can be due to retinal degeneration and retinitis pigmentosa.

83 Laurence-Moon-Biedl. Hypogonadism in an adolescent. Note the presence of testicles, partial scrotal development but microphallus.

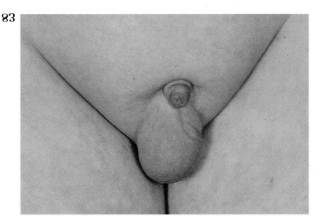

Alström syndrome

This very rare syndrome is characterised by blindness in infancy due to retinal degeneration, followed by the development of obesity, cataracts and nerve deafness in childhood. Diabetes mellitus with insulin resistance and chronic, progressive nephropathy appear, often in the child's teenage years or even later. Other features which are usually present include acanthosis nigricans, baldness, hyperuricaemia, hypertriglyceridaemia, scoliosis and hyperostosis frontalis interna. Hypogonadism is found in the males but not in the females. In the males there is primary testicular failure with small testicles, low serum testosterone levels and high gonadotrophins. Alström differs from Laurence-Moon-Biedl syndrome, which it superficially resembles, in that there is an absence of mental retardation and digital anomalies in the former, whereas nerve deafness, diabetes mellitus and chronic nephropathy are rare in the latter.

Kidney histology in Alström's syndrome has shown diffuse thickening of glomerular sclerosis, tubular atrophy and interstitial fibrosis. Membrane thickening and hyalinisation have also been found in the testes and skin. An interesting feature of this syndrome is that the obesity may regress as the patient ages. The syndrome would appear to be transmitted as an autosomal recessive (ref. 22).

There are many other extremely rare syndromes associated with obesity. **Carpenter syndrome** is associated with mental retardation, male hypogonadism, acrocephaly, polydactyly and syndactyly. **Cohen syndrome** has microcephaly, severe mental retardation, short stature and facial abnormalities (ref. 23). **Morgagni-Stewart-Morel** is a combination of the syndromes described by Morel and Morgagni. In **Morel syndrome** there is obesity, hyperostosis of the frontal bone, headache, nervous disturbance and a tendency to mental disorder. In **Morgagni syndrome** obesity is associated with internal frontal hyperostosis and virilism.

84 Hyperostosis Frontalis Interna. This is a common condition but is also one of the features in Alström's syndrome. Note the bone abnormality over the frontal region.

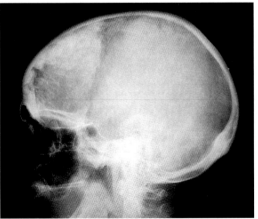

84

DIDMOAD syndrome

This syndrome is not uncommon. DIDMOAD is an acronym for the major features of the syndrome, namely diabetes insipidus, diabetes mellitus, optic atrophy and deafness. Friedreich's ataxia, cerebellar ataxia, bladder and ureter atonia, polyneuritis, retinitis pigmentosa and hypogonadism are other occasional features of the syndrome. Most are associated with mild obesity.

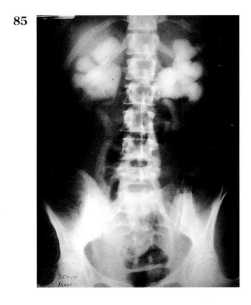

85 DIDMOAD. Intravenous pyelogram showing gross ureteric dilatation.

86 Optic atrophy is a characteristic feature of DIDMOAD syndrome. Mild obesity is often found.

Mental retardation and physical disability

Many patients with disorders producing mental retardation (e.g. Down's) or just physical disability can develop obesity even though the disorders involved are not directly the cause of the weight problem.

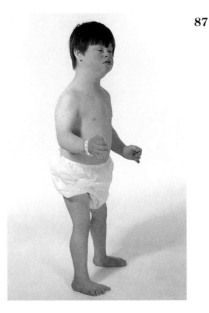

87 Down's syndrome. Mentally retarded children and adults do tend to be obese.

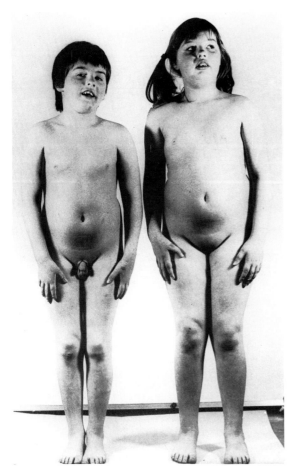

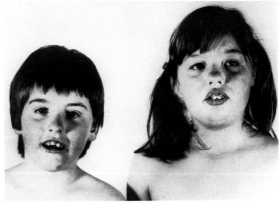

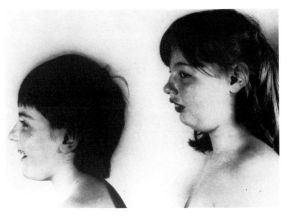

88 Cohen syndrome. The two patients are siblings. There are distinctive facial features, namely prominent nasal bridge, downward slanting palpebral fissures, open mouth appearance due to a short philtrum, prominent upper central incisors and retrogenia. The palate is usually high and narrow and the teeth irregularly spaced. There is microcephaly, mental retardation, short stature and cubitus valgus. The truncal obesity appears in mid childhood. Hypotonia, epilepsy, hyperextensible joints and delayed puberty are also often found in this rare syndrome. One must point out that the variablity of this disorder is wide and even obesity has not been reported in all cases (ref. 23).

4 Endocrine Causes

Hypothalamic obesity

Damage to the hypothalamus has been associated with massive gains in weight. The major difference between hypothalamic and essential obesity is that insulin levels are higher and hyperphagia is definitely present in the former.

In the experimental animal hyperinsulinaemia occurs within the first few days after lesions have been placed in the rat's ventromedial hypothalamus, well before there is any increase in body fat, and this rise in insulin cannot be prevented by controlling food intake. Bilateral section of the vagus nerve below the diaphragm abolishes the hyperphagia of the hypothalamic lesioned rodent and weight then returns to normal. The same experiment in genetically obese rodents does not modify their hyperphagia suggesting a specific role for the vagus nerve in experimental hypothalamic obesity.

Recent work in rodents has indicated that insulin-sensitive neurones, in or about the ventromedial hypothalamic area, play an important role in the integrations of dietary intake and sympathetic activity. Stimulation of this area activates interscapular brown fat thermogenesis and therefore lesions in this area may well reduce energy expenditure in the hypothalamic lesioned animal.

Hypothalamic obesity in man is associated with temperature regulating abnormalities. Although some have reported similar resting metabolic rates in hypothalamic and essential obesity in man, free living energy expenditure measurements have yet to be done and thus it is not possible to say conclusively whether an energy expenditure abnormality is present or otherwise. An abnormality of this type could explain why vagotomy has not been successful in treating such patients, as would have been predicted from animal studies. Although endocrine disorders of the gonadotrophic, thyroid and adrenal axis are often found in such patients, profound obesity can result without such impairment. A lack of growth hormone reducing muscle mass, and hence possibly energy expenditure, may play a role in some.

Table 17. Hypothalamic/Endocrine Causes

Hypothalamic

Trauma	
Inflammation —	Meningitis
	Encephalitis
	Tuberculosis
	Syphilis
Infiltration —	Sarcoidosis
	Histiocytosis X
Tumours —	Craniopharyngioma
	Astrocytoma
Leukaemic leucodystrophy	

Endocrine

Hypothalamus/ Pituitary —	Hyperprolactinaemia
	Kallman's syndrome
	Panhypopituitarism
	Growth hormone failure
	Laron Dwarf
	Cushing's disease
Thyroid —	Cretin
	Primary and secondary hypothyroidism
	Rarely thyrotoxicosis
Adrenal —	Cushing's syndrome
Ovary —	Polycystic ovarian syndrome
	Post-menopausal
	Turner's syndrome
Testes —	Primary hypogonadal
	Klinefelter's syndrome
	Sertoli Cell only syndrome
	Noonan's syndrome

The causes of hypothalamic obesity are trauma, inflammatory and infiltratory diseases, drugs and tumours. Obesity due to **trauma** tends to occur in the more active years of life (ages 5-40 years) and affects both sexes. It is reported that weight gain usually ceases after six months and some patients can then return to their original weight.

Inflammatory and infiltrative diseases of the hypothalamus which produce obesity include meningitis, syphilis, arachnoiditis, encephalitis, tuberculosis, sarcoidosis and histiocytosis X.

Somnolence and abnormalities of endocrine function are frequently associated with the causative disease.

Patients with **solid tumours** in the region of the hypothalamus represent the largest group of patients with hypothalamic obesity. Craniopharyngioma is the most common lesion associated with hypothalamic obesity occurring in over 50% of cases. Obesity is noted especially when the tumour involves the basal hypothalamus injuring the ventromedial nuclear areas. Other causes are rare and include pituitary adenomas, gliomas, hamartomas, epidermoid lesions, cysts, meningioma and chordomas.

Leukaemia has been recognised as a cause of hypothalamic obesity. In acute lymphatic leukaemia over 80% of those who suffer a CNS relapse die and many of those who live suffer severe handicap. A leukoencephalopathy has been recently described following therapy for leukaemic brain involvement. It appears to be the result not only of leukaemic infiltration of the brain, but also the effects of therapy involving both cranial irradiation and intrathecal and systemic methotrexate. The patients develop fits, deteriorating cerebral function, short stature, scanty hair growth and obesity. The condition is progressive and the patient often deteriorates to a demented state.

89

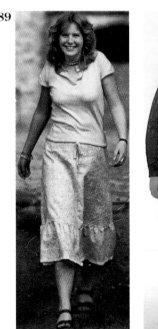

90

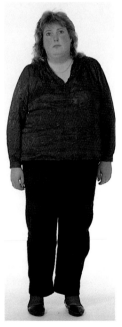

89 & 90 Histiocytosis X. The patient shown prior to diagnosis (**89**) and some years later (**90**) during the course of the disease. Her weight more than doubled on developing histiocytosis X. She initially developed diabetes insipidus with later panhypopituitarism. Both lung and bone infiltration have occurred.

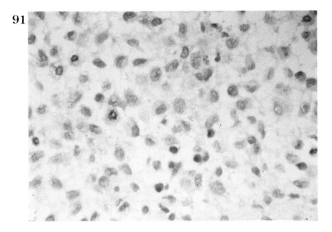

91 Histiocytosis X pathology. Characterised by the presence of many macrophages, some multinucleated forming giant cells and eosinophils. Predominance of the latter originally gave the alternative descriptive name 'eosinophilic granuloma'.

92 Eosinophilic granuloma involving the glenoid area of the scapula.

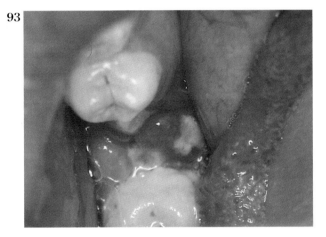

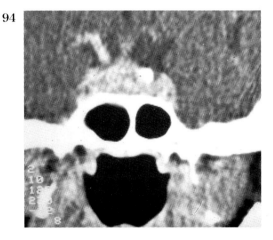

93 Histiocytosis X. Bony involvement of the mandible and maxilla can be a presenting feature as in this patient where the lesion produced a mouth ulcer.

94 Sarcoidosis. This condition, when it involves the hypothalamus, can produce obesity. Note the thickened pituitary stalk.

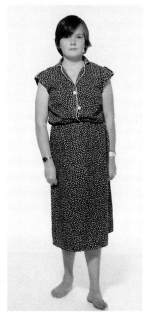

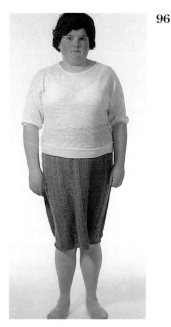

95 & 96 Craniopharyngioma. The patient at diagnosis (**95**) and some years later (**96**) when the condition had recurred, necessitating a second cranial operation. This patient intially required growth hormone but when this ceased her weight rapidly increased by over 20 kg.

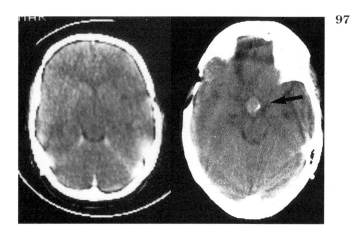

97 CAT brain scan of craniopharyngioma (arrow) on the right compared to a normal patient's scan on the left.

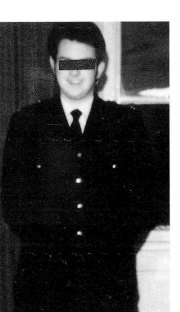

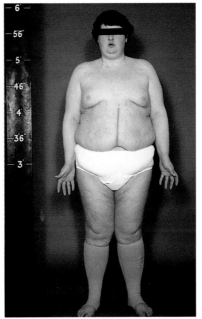

98 & 99 Craniopharyngioma. Pictures show the patient before diagnosis (**98**) and some years later (**99**) after the craniopharyngioma had been treated. Note the massive obesity. Abdominal scar was the result of an attempt to treat his obesity by truncal vagotomy which resulted in very little weight loss.

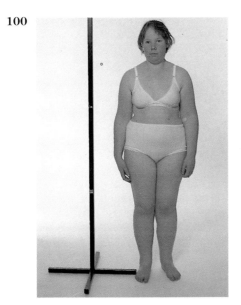

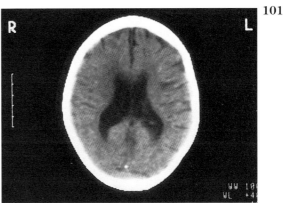

100 Leukaemic leucodystrophy. Mild obesity in this patient who was previously treated for acute lymphoblastic leukaemia with brain infiltration by irradiation and intrathecal methotrexate. Some years after successful therapy she developed gradual mental impairment and began to put on weight.

101 Brain CAT scan in leukaemic leucodystrophy of patient in **100**, showing dilated ventricles and brain atrophy.

Endocrine causes of obesity

Idiopathic obesity is generally associated with acceleration in growth. Obese children who are tall for their age rarely suffer from any endocrine abnormality. If the obesity extends into the second decade, then puberty begins early and there is advanced skeletal development which results in obese children being no taller as adults than would be expected from their genetic potential. Endocrine causes of obesity, however, are usually associated with growth impairment. One must emphasise that endocrine disorders are extremely rare causes of obesity, perhaps present in less than 0.1% of all overweight children. **Growth hormone failure** in children is associated with variable degrees of truncal obesity which usually regresses rapidly when growth hormone therapy is given. Mild obesity can also be a feature of the Laron-type dwarfism in which there is a failure to generate somatomedins and profound resistance to growth hormone. These children have high serum growth hormone levels and do not respond to exogenous growth hormone therapy. Their puberty is delayed and final height is rarely in excess of 130 cm. This condition occurs mainly in Jewish families, where both sexes can be affected, and is probably transmitted as a recessive trait.

Hypothalamic and pituitary pathology, which produce panhypopitutarism, can present with obesity, especially if adrenal reserves are not completely depleted. Frequently, the obesity is associated with hypogonadism, hypothyroidism and poor growth, as first reported by Fröhlich in his original case of a craniopharyngioma pressing upon the hypothalamus. Often such patients are called fat Fröhlich dwarfs. Nevertheless, most boys, in whom the diagnosis of Fröhlich's syndrome is entertained, are in fact suffering from essential obesity and the prepubertal genitalia are buried in a pubic pad of fat.

The clinical impression is that **hyperprolactinaemia** is often found in overweight and obese women. It is doubtful that this is a true association since one study suggested that obesity was not more prevalent in women with hyperprolactinaemia. A raised prolactin in men is often associated with a large, aggressive, pituitary tumour and obesity is more likely to be present not necessarily due to the raised prolactin itself but to the reduction in other hormones, especially coincidental hypogonadism and

Table 18.	Clinical Features of Hypothyroidism
General —	Lack of energy
	Weight gain
	Intolerance of cold
	Poor memory
Dermatological —	Dry skin
	Dry hair
	Loss of lateral eyebrows
	Bloated appearance
	Myxoedematous skin turgor
Cardiovascular —	Bradycardia
	Pericardial effusion
	Angina
	Cardiac failure
Gastrointestinal —	Acid regurgitation
	Constipation
Neuromuscular —	Muscle pains and weakness
	Carpal tunnel syndrome
	Deafness
	Hoarse voice
	Cerebellar ataxia
	Delayed relaxation of tendon reflexes
	Depression, psychosis
Reproduction —	Infertility
	Menorrhagia
	Galactorrhoea
Haematological —	Mild anaemia—macrocytosis without B_{12} or folate deficiency

hypothyroidism. Males often present with advanced disease and visual impairment whereas women present early due to menstrual abnormalities, infertility and galactorrhoea.

Hypothyroidism leads to weight gain due in part to a reduction by as much as 40% of the basal metabolic rate. There is also a change in body composition with a decrease in lean body mass, increase in tissue mucopolysaccharides and fluid retention. Clinical features of this condition are shown in **Table 18**. Clinicians often assume, as do patients, that treating hypothyroidism will result in a long-term reduction in body weight. However, after an initial short lived weight reduction due to loss of fluid, weight is often regained. In 25 hypothyroid, female, adult patients with a mean initial weight of 68.5 kg, weight loss after one year of thyroxine therapy averaged only 0.6 kg..

In those who are markedly obese thyroxine therapy for hypothyroidism may result in eventual weight gain, emphasising the underlying obesity problem.

It is important to emphasise that the clinical signs of hypothyroidism in newborns can be subtle and less than 5% of affected infants found on screening tests were suspected of hypothyroidism by prior clinical evaluation. Only a minority present with the classic cretin appearance. Early diagnosis is essential for, if delayed, there is a greater risk of mental retardation and neurological damage such as lack of co-ordination ataxia, spastic diplegia, hypotonia and strabismus.

Thyrotoxicosis is usually associated with profound weight loss, although there are some cases where the disease is associated with weight gain. This is seen especially in overweight, younger women. Obese individuals are just as prone as the rest of the population to the development of goitres, thyrotoxicosis and Graves' Eye disease. Such individuals may present with periorbital oedema, conjunctival inflammation (chemosis) or even congestive ophthalmopathy. It is important to recognise this in the obese and an unexpected weight loss may be an important signal to the diagnosis. Such patients may also develop localised myxoedema which commonly affects the pretibial region, although other parts of the body, determined by local trauma or pressure, may be involved. When this involves the lower legs of those with already obese limbs it may not at first be recognised for what it is. There are several forms of localised (pretibial) myxoedema, namely a nodular form, which can mimic erythema nodosum and come and go, a sheet-like form, with non-pitting oedema, coarse thickening of the skin and violaceous discolouration, and finally a warty form, with gross overgrowth of the skin and subcutaneous tissue.

Weight gain with the treatment of the thyrotoxicosis can be appreciable and is similar in the three modalities of therapy, namely drugs (carbimazole), radioactive iodine and partial thyroidectomy. Average weight gains of 5.4, 7.4 and 6.3 kg respectively have been observed one year after therapy, with about 60% of the increase in weight occurring in the first three months. It would appear that those who are most obese gain the most weight.

Pseudohypoparathyroidism comprises a

Table 19. Features of Pseudohypoparathyroidism	
Hypocalcaemia produces —	Tetany (65%) Fits (65%) Cramps (40%) Laryngeal spasm Paraesthesiae

Other features —	Subcutaneous and basal calcification (due to hyperphosphataemia) (60%)
	Cataracts (35%)
	Mental defects (10%)
	Skeletal—short metacarpals (70%)
	  short metatarsals (40%)
	  stocky, overweight (50-70%)
	  bone density increased (15%)
	  or decreased (15%)
	  thickened calvaria (20%)

spectrum of disorders characterised by the clinical and biochemical consequences of peripheral parathyroid hormone resistance associated with skeletal abnormalities. These are summarised in **Table 19**. Fifty to 70% of such patients have a stocky habitus, some being moderately obese.

In this syndrome there appears to be a hormone receptor dysfunction. The hormone receptor and adenyl cyclase are linked by membrane regulatory proteins in the cell membrane called N or G proteins. In pseudohypoparathyroidism there appears to be a defect of these proteins. This membrane protein dysfunction may extend to other hormone receptors as abnormalities in secretion and effects of thyrotrophin, prolactin, gonadotrophin, vasopressin, glucagon and insulin have been reported. The variability of the end organ defect probably accounts for the variations in this disorder. For instance, some may have renal resistance to parathyroid hormone whereas the bones are responsive, resulting in osteitis fibrosa cystica as seen in hyperparathyroidism and others have normal renal responsiveness but resistance in the bone. Partial forms of parathyroid resistance have also been reported. Pseudohypoparathyroidism is often familial and an X-linked inheritance has been suggested, based on lack of well documented cases of male to male transmission.

Table 20. Major Causes of the Features of Cushing's Syndrome
• Iatrogenic due to steroid therapy
• Pituitary tumour producing excess ACTH (Cushing's disease)
• Ectopic ACTH secretion (mainly carcinoma of lung)
• Adrenal adenoma or carcinoma
• Chronic alcohol abuse (pseudo-Cushing's).

Table 21. Clinical Features of Cushing's Syndrome	
Cardinal signs —	Proximal myopathy
	Chemosis
	Thin skin
	Frontal balding (in women)
	Osteoporosis (early onset)
Other signs —	Acne
	Hirsutism
	Buffalo hump
	Truncal obesity
	Purple striae
	Fat-filled supraclavicular fossae
	Bruising
	Oedema
	Hypotonia
	Kyphosis
	Pathological fractures
	Thirst
	Polyuria
	Glycosuria
	Diabetes mellitus
	Amenorrhoea
	Depression
	Growth retardation (in children)
	Bacterial infections
	Fungal infections

Pseudo-pseudohypoparathyroidism was originally coined for patients showing the typical phenotypic features of pseudohypoparathyroidism without the metabolic abnormalities. It is of interest that the mothers of girls with pseudohypoparathyroidism have been reported to show pseudo-pseudohypoparathyroidism. Some of the latter can . exhibit subtle signs of hormone resistance such as mildly elevated serum parathyroid hormone levels despite normal urinary cyclic AMP responses to exogenous parathyroid hormone infusion. This raises difficulties in explaining the genetic basis of pseudo-pseudohypoparathyroidism which are as yet unresolved.

Idiopathic hypoparathyroidism is not specifically associated with obesity, although in some, associated hypogonadism and hypothyroidism may result in a weight problem. This rare disease can also be associated with chronic mucocutaneous moniliasis due to a defect in cellular immunity, alopecia areata and vitiligo.

Cushing's syndrome results from an excess output of adrenal glucocorticoids, notably cortisol. There are a number of causes as outlined in **Table 20**.

The clinical features of this condition are shown in **Table 21**. Many of the features such as obesity, hypertension, oedema, hirsutism, diabetes mellitus, depression and facial plethora are often seen in idiopathic obesity and therefore diagnosis can be difficult unless the clinician considers the possibility of Cushing's. There are certain cardinal signs which aid in the diagnosis, namely proximal myopathy, thin skin, conjunctival oedema (chemosis), frontal balding (in women) and early onset osteoporosis. Striae are not diagnostic, often being seen in an obese person who rapidly puts on weight. Many patients with Cushing's syndrome whom I have seen have not had any striae whatsoever. The obesity is always truncal with thin arms and legs due to muscle wasting, associated with a plethoric face and fat-filled supraclavicular fossae. In the case of children the obesity is associated with marked growth retardation and osteoporosis. Some patients (but not all) also exhibit hypokalaemic alkalosis. Diagnosis of this condition biochemically in an obese patient is best done by measuring 24 hr urinary-free cortisol. Often in obese subjects urinary-free cortisol is at the upper limit of normal or even borderline elevated. In such a situation a 1 mg overnight dexamethasone test or, better still, a low dose, prolonged dexamethasone test (2 mg per day for 2 days) will clarify the situation. In the overnight test 1 mg tablet of dexamethasone is taken by the patient at midnight. The next morning a 9 a.m., venous sample is taken for plasma cortisol. A normal response is suppression of cortisol to less than 150 mmol/l. Anything higher than this would lead one to suspect Cushing's. Nevertheless, one must emphasise that if clinical suspicion is strong, a normal overnight suppression test should not be taken as totally excluding the condition and in such circumstances the patient should be admitted for more extensive hospital investigations. The condition is too dangerous to leave since the five-year, untreated mortality is about 50%, with deaths from cardiovascular disease, infection and suicide.

Treatment of this disease depends on the cause. For pituitary tumours, surgery or radioactive Yttrium-90 implantation is effective. For an adenoma, surgical removal is curative but for an ectopic source, if the primary is inoperable or not found, bilateral adrenalectomy is necessary. If bilateral adrenalectomy is performed for a pituitary tumour, a favourite treatment in the past, then the tumour remains in the pituitary fossa, expands and eventually causes **Nelson's syndrome** with excess pigmentation, eventual visual failure and cavernous sinus involvement. Frequently chronic alcohol excess can mimic Cushing's syndrome and is often called 'Pseudo-Cushing's'. The signs can be similar and urinary-free cortisol is elevated. Alcohol removal is curative.

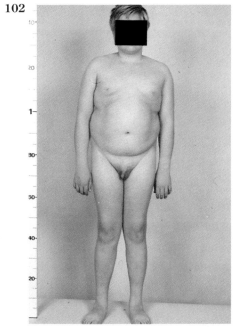

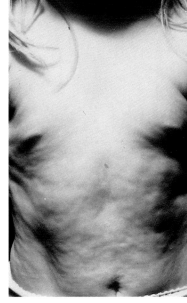

102 **Growth hormone deficiency** produced mild obesity in this boy. Note the fatty gynaecomastia.

103 **Growth hormone deficiency.** The fat has a special, marbled appearance quite unlike that seen in essential obesity.

104

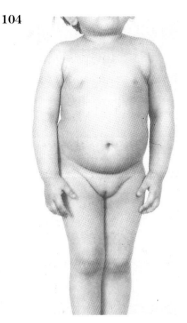

105

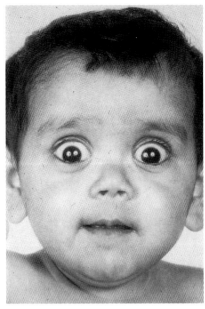

104 Laron dwarf. The hands and feet are small for the body size. Subcutaneous fat is well developed despite the fact that these children appear to eat less than their normal siblings. Voice is often high pitched but intelligence is normal.

105 Laron dwarf. The facial bones grow more slowly than the cranial vault resulting in a bulging forehead, small face, saddle nose and a staring appearance. Note also the slow hair growth with deep temporal recession.

106

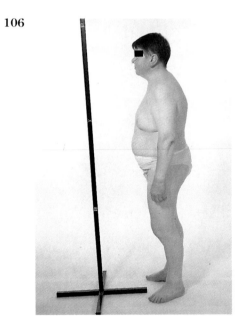

107

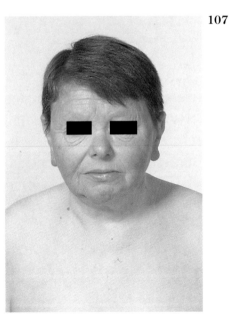

106 Panhypopituitarism. Note the central obesity, gynaecomastia and short stature in this middle-aged man. CT scan showed a partially empty pituitary sella.

107 Panhypopituitarism. Facial view of patient in **106** shows an absence of facial hair, fine, unwrinkled skin, thinning of eyebrows and dry hair. Although in his mid-forties he had the facial appearance of an elderly man.

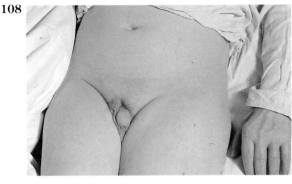

108 Panhypopituitarism. This patient with panhypopituitarism had mild obesity, a marked decrease in pubic hair and shrunken testicles. Axillary and facial hair was absent.

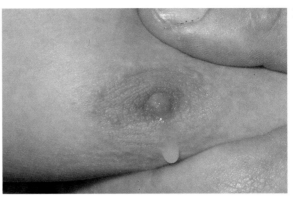

109 Galactorrhoea and gynaecomastia in a young obese man with a prolactin secreting pituitary tumour.

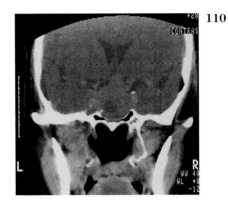

110 CAT scan of pituitary shows the pituitary tumour extending downwards into the sphenoid sinus and laterally and upwards into the hypothalamic region.

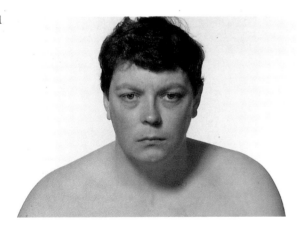

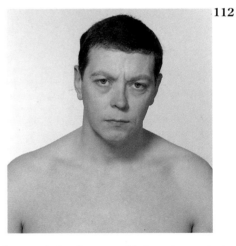

111 & 112 Prolactinoma. The patient on presentation weighed 100 kg (**111**) and had a raised serum prolactin (28000 mu/l) but normal serum thyroxine, testosterone and cortisol response to hypoglycaemia. Following transphenoidal surgery, external radiotherapy and bromocriptine therapy, with thyroxine and hydrocortisone replacement, he lost 20 kg in weight without any specific diet and with no effort. Prior to therapy he was unable to lose weight. Note the thinner face and loss of fat over the shoulders.

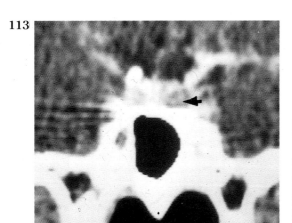

113 Microprolactinoma. Most women with hyperprolactinaemia do not show massive pituitary enlargement. Some show a microprolactinoma seen here (arrowed) as a low density area. This was later confirmed when it was removed at surgery.

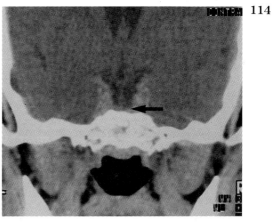

114 Hyperprolactinaemia. This obese woman with hyperprolactinaemia had a partially empty sella. Note the pituitary stalk extending to a small rim of pituitary tissue (arrowed) at the base of pituitary fossa.

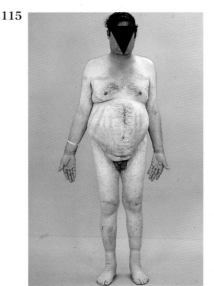

115 Cushing's syndrome showing the classical features of truncal obesity, wasted legs and arms with proximal muscle weakness, abdominal and thoracic striae, lower leg oedema and bruising.

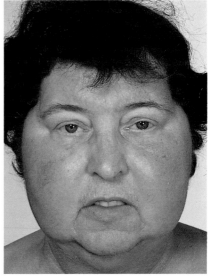

116 Cushing's syndrome showing typical plethoric, full, rounded face, glistening eyes due to conjunctival oedema, moderate hirsutism and filling out of the supraclavicular fat pads.

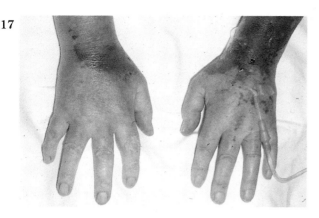

117 Thin skin in Cushing's syndrome. Note the extensive bruising brought about by venepuncture.

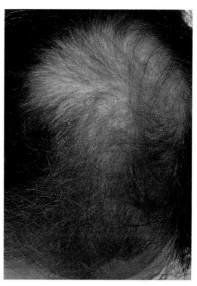

118 Frontal and vortex balding. This is often a feature in women with Cushing's syndrome.

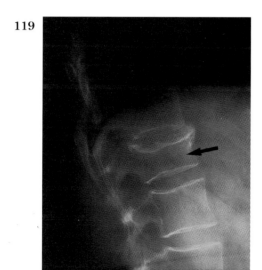

119 Osteoporosis is often marked in Cushing's syndrome. Note the partially collapsed vertebrum (arrowed). Collapse of a vertebrum in the thoracic spine produces the kyphosis often seen in Cushing's.

120 Oral candidiasis in a patient with Cushing's disease.

121 Pityriasis versicolor. Fungal and yeast infections (**120**) are a common problem in Cushing's syndrome. The scaly rash appears as circular patches.

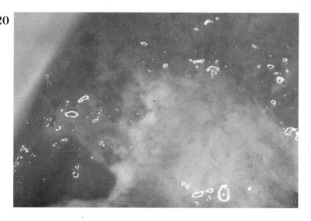

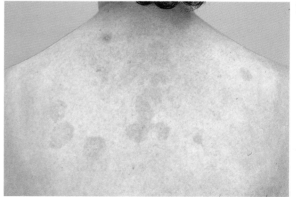

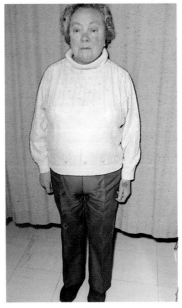 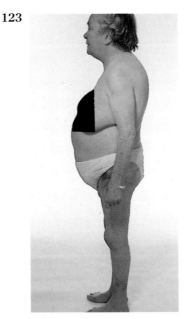 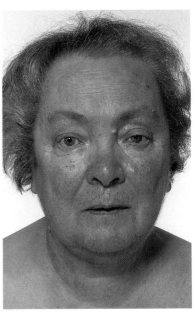

122　Cushing's disease. This patient attended the diabetic clinical where her hypertension was a problem. Hypertension is seen in nearly 50% of type II diabetic patients and so this combination did not alert the physician until control of her blood pressure necessitated hospital admission.

123　Cushing's disease. Unclothed the patient in **122** showed the typical appearance of Cushing's disease. Note the marked truncal obesity, wasted arms and legs and kyphosis. She had thin skin and proximal myopathy but no striae, emphasising that the latter is not pathognomic of Cushing's.

124　Facial appearance of Cushing's patient in **122** and **123**. Note the plethoric cheeks, hirsutism and temporal hair recession.

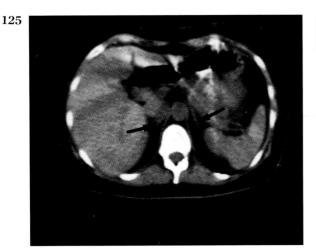 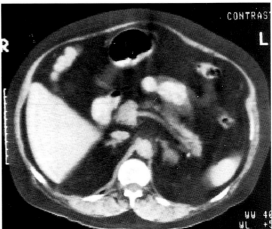

125 & 126　Adrenal CAT scans. 125 shows normal adrenals (arrows). **126** shows hyperplastic adrenal tissue. Pituitary tumour was later removed by transphenoidal surgery curing the patient of her Cushing's disease, diabetes and hypertension.

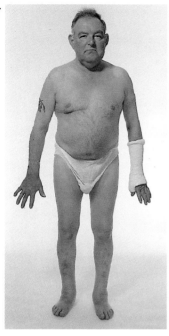 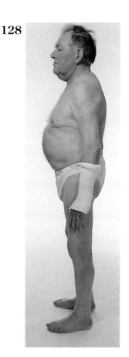 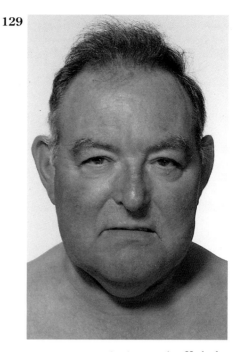

127–129 Cushing's syndrome. The patient shown in **127** to **129** initially presented in 1988 having fallen out of his lorry fracturing his left arm. His difficulty climbing into the cab of his lorry was due to proximal myopathy. He had truncal obesity, no striae, thin skin and a Cushingoid face.

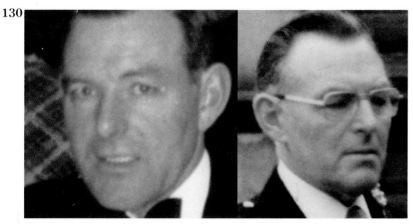

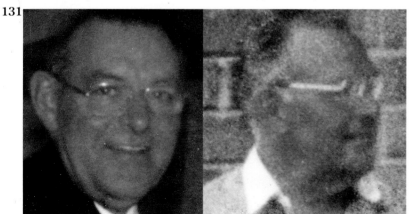

130 & 131 Development of Cushing's syndrome. Family album pictures of patient in-**127** to **129** taken in 1974, 1978, 1981 and 1987. These photographs indicate that his Cushing's developed gradually from about 1981.

132 **Adrenal scan** of patient in **127** to **131** showed an extensive, right adrenal mass (thick arrow) with an atrophic, left adrenal gland (thin arrow).

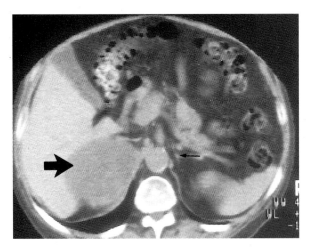

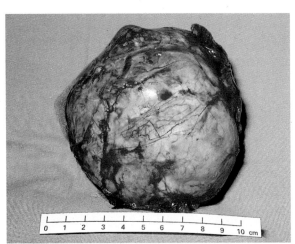

133 **Adrenal adenoma** removed from patient with CAT picture (shown in **132**) was the size of a large grapefruit. This operation cured his Cushing's syndrome.

134 **Post-operative**. Compare this picture, taken after the adrenal adenoma was removed, with that taken pre-operatively in **129**. Note the change in facial appearance even though he weighed only 2 kg less than when he had Cushing's syndrome.

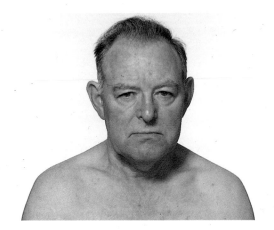

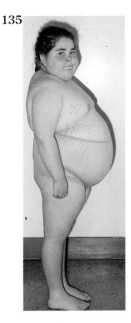
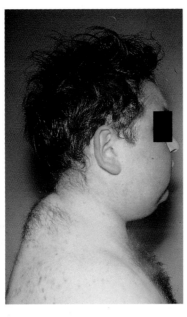
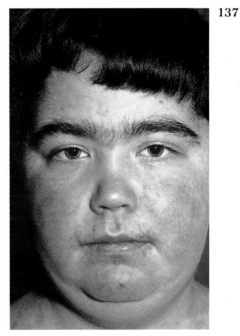

135 Cushing's disease in a young girl. Again note the extensive, truncal obesity and facial appearance. There is also reduced growth which contrasts with the presentation in simple obesity where growth is often accelerated.

136 Buffalo hump in this boy with Cushing's, together with overlying whorl of hair and associated acne.

137–140 Cushing's disease in a young boy before (**137** and **138**) and after treatment (**139** and **140**) with 90-Yttrium interstitial pituitary implantation. Note the remarkable change in body and facial habitus that occurs once this disease is cured.

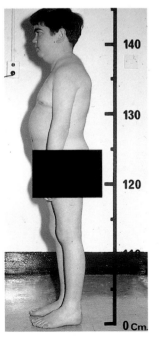
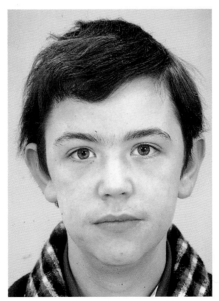
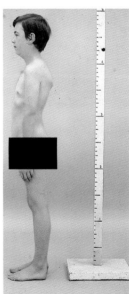

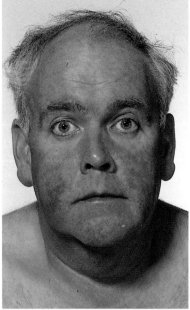

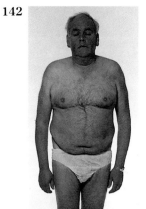

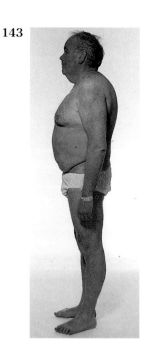

141–143 Pseudo Cushing's due to alcohol. This patient's high urinary-free cortisol levels were reduced to normal after one week's cessation of alcohol. Note the truncal distribution of fat and plethoric face with parotid enlargement.

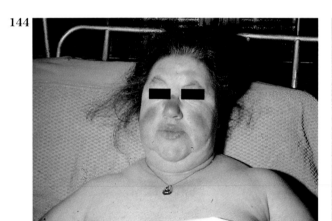

144 Myxoedema. Lethargic, somnolent women with dry skin, dry hair and 'strawberries and cream' complexion. Note the malar flush and 'cream' complexion due to raised levels of carotene.

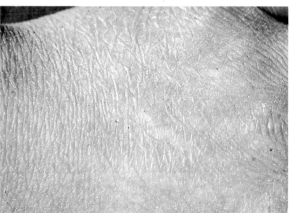

145 Dry skin in a patient with myxoedema.

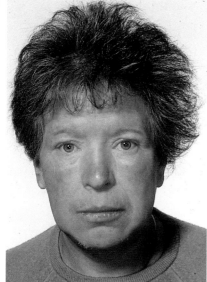

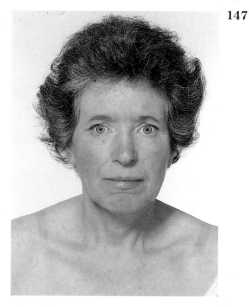

146 & 147 Myxoedema. Marked change in facial appearance before (**146**) and after treatment with thyroxine replacement therapy (**147**).

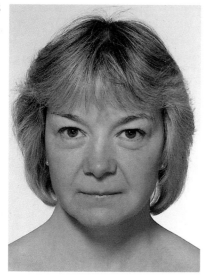

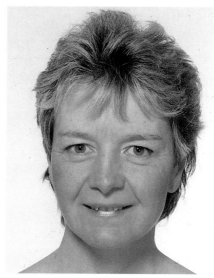

148 & 149 Myxoedema. Again a marked change before (**148**) and after treatment (**147**). Note how much more lively the treated face appears.

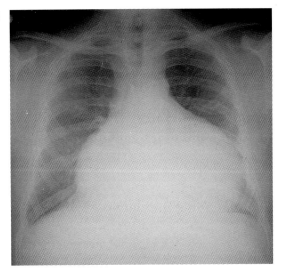

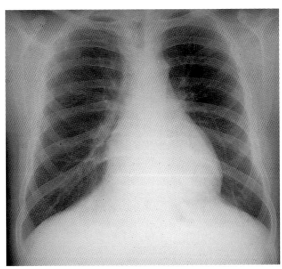

150 & 151 Pericardial effusion can develop in longstanding myxoedema. Note the widened heart shadow due to pericardial fluid (**150**) confirmed by echocardiography. Slow increase in thyroxine replacement over many months resulted in resolution of the pericardial fluid (10 months in this case) (**151**).

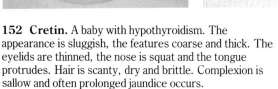

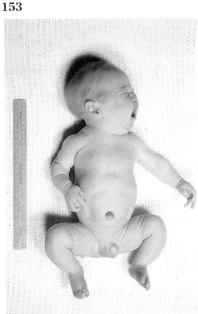

152 Cretin. A baby with hypothyroidism. The appearance is sluggish, the features coarse and thick. The eyelids are thinned, the nose is squat and the tongue protrudes. Hair is scanty, dry and brittle. Complexion is sallow and often prolonged jaundice occurs.

153 Cretin. The abdomen is pot-bellied and and umbilical hernia is common.

154 Treated hypothyroidism in the patient shown in **152** and **153** at age of two years.

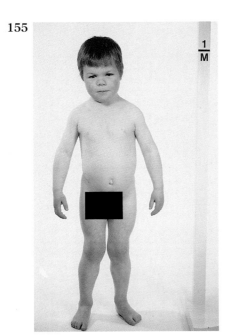

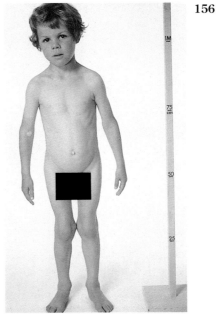

155 & 156 Hypothyroid boy before and after treatment with thyroxine. Note the coarse features with typical myxoedematous facies (**155**) and the transformation on treatment with thyroxine (**156**).

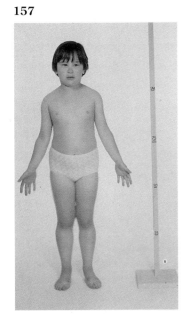

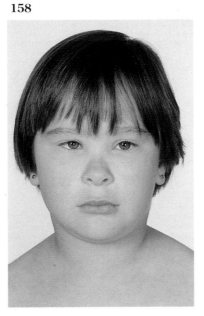

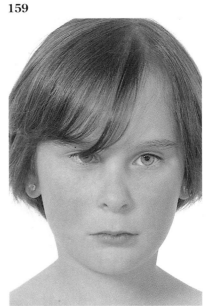

157–159 Hypothyroid girl before (**157** and **158**) and after thyroxine therapy (**159**).

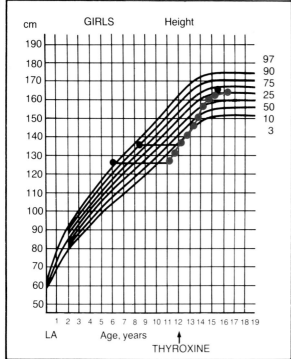

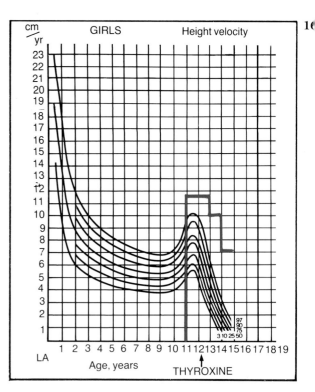

160 Growth chart of the patient in **157** to **159** shows that before therapy growth was retarded (red dots) with delayed bone age (black dots). On thyroxine, growth and bone age rapidly caught up, equalling chronological age at 15 years.

161 Growth velocity. Pictorial presentation showing marked improvement of growth velocity on thyroxine.

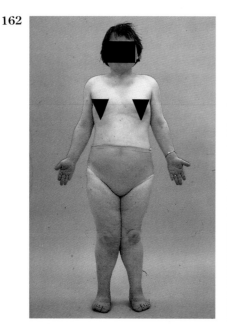

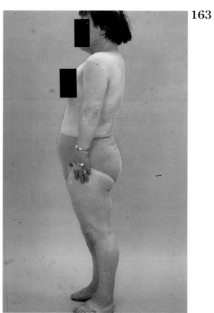

162 & 163 Pseudohypoparathyroidism. This patient, then 44 years of age, had long-standing hypocalcaemia, epilepsy and was of short stature. She had a stocky build with rounded face.

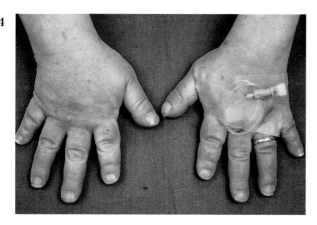

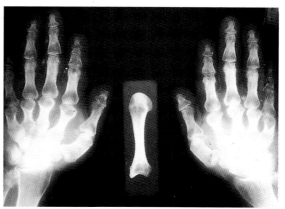

164 Pseudohypoparathyroidism. The hands (and also the feet) are small and stubby in this patient.

165 Radiology of the hands of patient in **164** to show that the stubby nature of the hands is due to shortening of all five metacarpals. Note also the subcutaneous calcification.

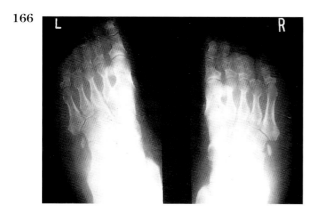

166

167

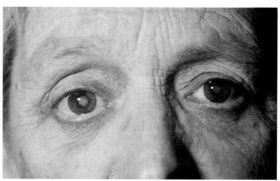

166 Radiology of feet of pseudohypoparathyroid patient. Note that all five metatarsals are shortened.

167 Cataracts in a pseudohypoparathyroid patient.

168

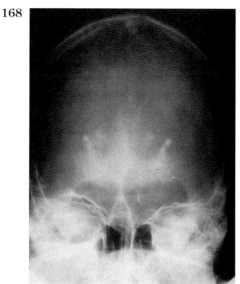

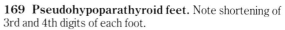

168 Basal ganglia calcification in pseudohypoparathyroidism.

169 Pseudohypoparathyroid feet. Note shortening of 3rd and 4th digits of each foot.

169

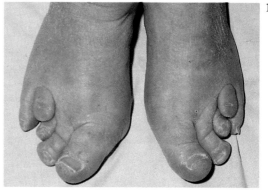

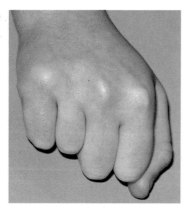

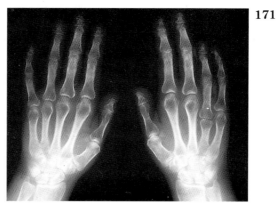

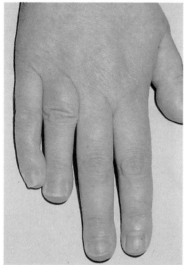

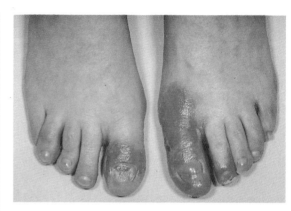

170 Pseudo-pseudohypoparathyroidism has similar phenotype to pseudohypoparathyroidism but patients are eucalcaemic. In this patient the fourth metacarpal is shortened, resulting in the absence of the 4th knuckle.

171 Hand radiology of patient in **170** confirming the shortened 4th metacarpal of the right hand.

172 Pseudo-pseudohypoparathyroidism. In this condition (and incidentally in pseudohypoparathyroidism also) the most usual feature is to find both the 4th and 5th fingers reduced due to shortening of the metacarpals concerned, as illustrated here.

173 Idiopathic hypoparathyroidism with chronic mucocutaneous moniliasis.

Gonadal

Ovary and testes

Males with hypogonadism of whatever cause tend to be obese, some more than others. The distribution of fat is of a female type, mainly involving the lower abdomen, hips and thighs.

Hypogonadal females tend to be less obese when accurate measurements are taken. One such example is the situation in **Turner's syndrome**. In 70% of cases this is due to an XO karyotype, the remainder having mosaic XO/XX forms or deletions of the short or long arm of an X chromosome. Streak gonads are present and patients are of short stature with a characteristic habitus and may have congenital heart lesions involving the left side of the heart and aorta. Although many patients with Turner's syndrome appear obese, when assessed by measurements of skinfold thickness this is often not significant. Turner's phenotype, **Noonan's syndrome**, also can occur in some females and males with a normal karyotype but with right-sided· heart lesions. The males are often hypogonadal with an overweight or obese habitus.

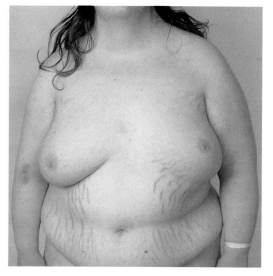

174

174 Turner's syndrome. Obesity such as this is not often a feature of this syndrome. Note the neck webbing. The striae did not indicate Cushing's. This patient has had ostrogen therapy to promote secondary sexual characteristics.

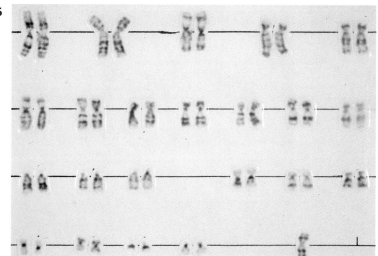

175 Chromosomes in Turner's syndrome showing only one X chromosome.

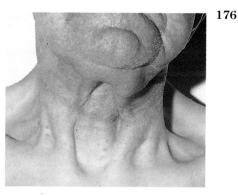

176

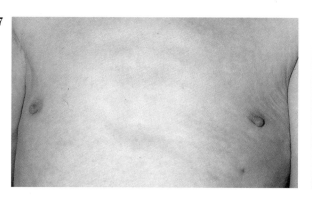

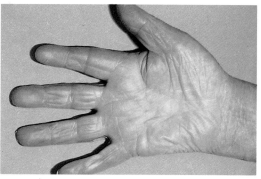

178

176–178 Noonan's syndrome. A hypogonadal, mildly obese man with a Turner's phenotype and pulmonary stenosis. Note the neck webbing (**176**), wide nipple spacing (**177**) and simian crease (**178**).

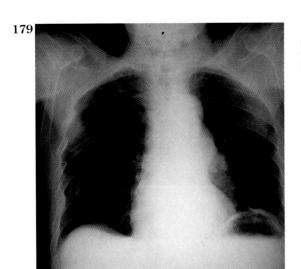

179 **Radiology of chest in Noonan's syndrome** showing pulmonary hypertension with prominent pulmonary vasculature at hilum, especially noticeable on the left side.

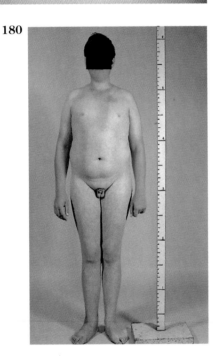

180 **Klinefelter's syndrome.** This hypogonadal boy was tall with a typical hypogonadal obesity distribution mainly affecting the abdomen, hips and thighs. His chromosome complete was 46 XXY.

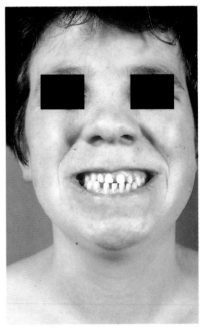

181 **Hypogonadotrophic hypogonadism** (Kallman's syndrome). Over half the patients have somatic abnormalities. This patient had typical hypogonadal obesity, lack of smell, depressed nasal bridge and abnormal dentition with widely-spaced teeth. These oro-facial abnormalities, icythosis, deafness, red-green blindness and cryptorchidism are all characteristic features of this condition.

5 Metabolic, Drug, Insulinoma and Hyperlipidaemia

Drugs

Diabetes mellitus therapy

Sulphonlyurea-type drugs used to treat non-insulin-type diabetes mellitus have been implicated in modest weight gain. This is not a feature of the use of the biguanide, **metformin**. The reason for this difference has yet to be explained as the resting metabolic rate is similar on both drugs if glycaemic control is comparable. Possibly the difference in glucose energy loss in the urine may be the explanation. On tightening diabetic control in **insulin**-dependent diabetes weight gain is often seen. Two factors at least account for this. The first is the reduction of the metabolic rate and the second, a reduction in glucose energy losses with tight glycaemic control.

Smoking

Cessation of **smoking** is also implicated in many with weight gain. Recent research shows that the catecholamines released by smoking one cigarette produce about 9 kcal (37 kj) of heat. Therefore, if a person stops smoking 20 cigarettes, energy intake must be reduced 180 kcals (0.74 MJ) to compensate or weight will otherwise be gained as this excess energy is not burnt off but stored as fat. Increased appetite on cessation of smoking also plays an important role.

Sex hormones

Oestrogen therapy, especially in the form of the **contraceptive pill**, is also associated with weight gain. This is due in part to the cessation of ovulation which then prevents the usual small rise in energy expenditure in the luteal phase. Water retention and altered appetite also play a role.

Alcohol

Alcohol usually produces weight gain due to the high energy content of most alcoholic beverages. In some people alcohol can induce pseudo-Cushing's as mentioned in Chapter 4.

Corticosteroids

Corticosteroids in doses above the physiological replacement level induce weight gain due to fat deposition by facilitating the action of insulin in promoting fatty acid uptake into adipose tissue. In higher dosages gluocorticoids induce the picture of iatrogenic Cushing's syndrome.

Table 22. Drugs Associated with Weight Gain
Insulin
Sulphonylurea
Oestrogen
Contraceptive pill
Alcohol
Corticosteroids
Cyproheptadine
Sodium valproate
Phenothiazines
Tricyclic antidepressants
Nonselective ß adrenergic blockers

182

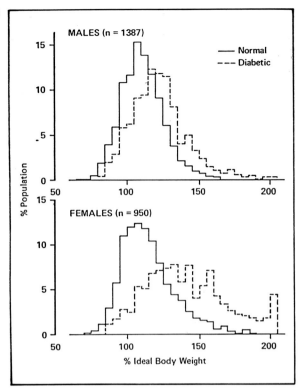

MALES (n = 1387)

— Normal
--- Diabetic

% Population

% Ideal Body Weight

FEMALES (n = 950)

182 Weight in type II diabetic patients at time of diagnosis is greater than that in the general non-diabetic population and this is especially marked in females. The data in **182** and **183** is derived from the UK Prospective Diabetic Study.

183 Weight change with hypoglycaemic therapy.
Initially the type II diabetic patients were on a diet alone for 3 months, hence the fall in weight initially from -3 to 0 months. As glycaemic control was poor, the patients were randomly allocated to sulphonylurea, insulin or metformin. Note that insulin and sulphonylurea produce somewhat similar rises in weight. In contrast, metformin produces little or no weight gain.

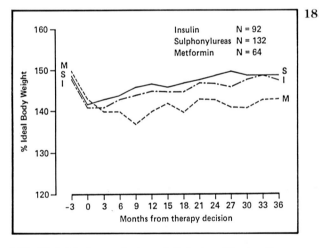

18

Insulin	N = 92
Sulphonylureas	N = 132
Metformin	N = 64

% Ideal Body Weight

Months from therapy decision

184

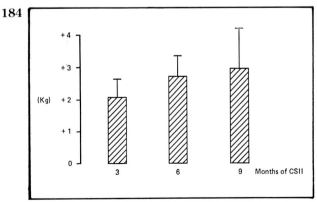

(Kg)

Months of CSII

184 Weight change in type I diabetes. Nine insulin dependent patients had their glycaemic control improved by changing their insulin therapy from twice daily injections to continuous subcutaneous insulin infusion (CSII). Weight gain was gradual (ref. 25).

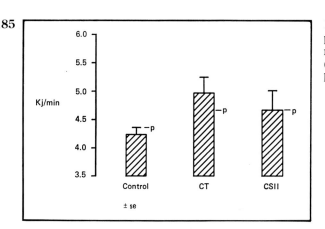

185 Resting metabolic rate. Weight gain in the patients in **185** was due to a reduction of resting metabolic rate to predicted levels (P) on CSII amounting to 90 kcal (374 Kj) per day, and to a decrease in urinary glucose losses (ref. 25).

186

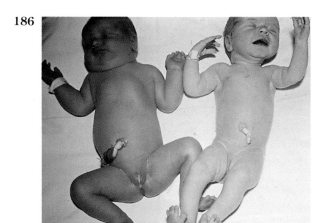

186 'Diabetic' baby. The baby on the left was born to a poorly controlled, diabetic mother and is compared to a baby born to a healthy mother on the right. The baby born to the diabetic mother is lethargic, heavier, fat deposition is increased and the viscera is enlarged but immature. Some 5% have congenital abnormalities and the baby is prone to respiratory distress and special unit care is initially required. The baby loses a considerable amount of weight but the progress after the initial few weeks of life is similar to that of other children.

187

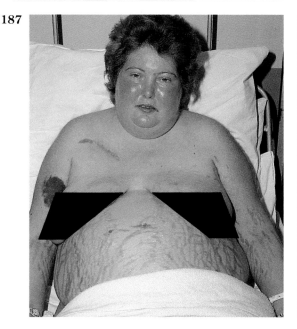

188

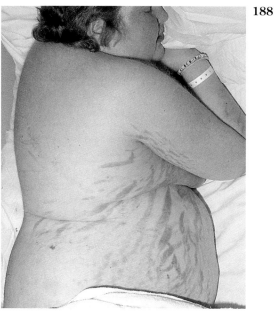

187 Corticosteroid excess produces a Cushingoid picture. Note the truncal obesity, reddened face and bruising on the right arm with multiple striae over the abdomen and even on the arms.

188 Corticosteroid excess showing voilaceous striae and truncal obesity.

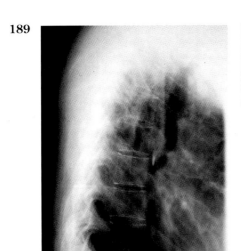

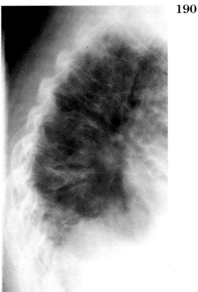

189 & 190 Corticosteroid induced osteoporosis.
189 illustrates the thoracic spine before corticosteroids. **190** is from the same patient on corticosteroids. Note the marked osteoporosis with collapse of the vertebrae producing kyphosis.

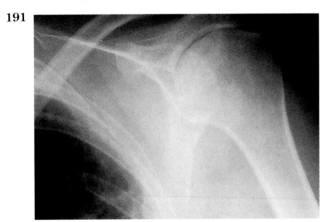

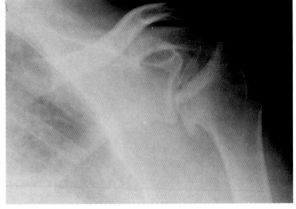

191 & 192 Corticosteroid induced ischaemic necrosis. 191 shows the earliest changes of ischaemic necrosis in the humeral head. **192** is from the same patient one year later, showing severe ischaemic necrotic collapse in the humeral head.

Insulinoma

This is a rare tumour, most frequently presenting in middle age with a higher incidence in women than men (ratio 3:2). The most common presentation is of sweating, palpitations, tremor, hunger and generalised weakness after an overnight fast or following exercise, which are relieved by food. If the patients recognise this they may increase their carbohydrate intake with consequent weight gain. The gain is variable. In some it is not seen at all and in most others it is modest. In one series of 60 cases one-fifth gained weight when symptomatic and at diagnosis 50% of males and females were overweight or distinctly obese. Eighty% of patients with insulinoma become hypoglycaemic after an overnight fast if three consecutive observations are made, but the proportion rises to 98% if fasting is continued for 48 hours and terminated by a spell of brisk exercise. A low, fasting, plasma-glucose value (e.g. 2.2. mmol/l) in the presence of an elevated plasma-insulin level is indicative of insulinoma. Blood glucose in healthy non-obese males rarely falls below 2.8 mmol/l with prolonged fasting but it may be lower (as much as 1.7 mmol/l) in healthy non-obese females and children. Nevertheless, in healthy individuals no symptoms occur and insulin levels are extremely low or indiscernible. Due possibly to episodic secretion of insulin by tumours and increased hepatic uptake, some rare cases have had hypoglycaemia with low plasma insulin levels. In such circumstances an amended insulin to glucose ratio may be useful (insulin uu/ml x 100 divided by plasma glucose in mg/dl-30). In non-obese individuals a value of 49 or less is considered normal.

Difficulty may arise in the obese who have elevated, fasting insulin levels due to insulin resistance and often healthy individuals may have values above 50. A useful rule of thumb is to note that fasting plasma-glucose is usually above 3 mmol/l in obese subjects without tumour, but always below this in obese patients with insulinoma.

Location of the tumour is not easy, the best technique being selective coeliac axis angiography in skilled hands, with an accuracy of 55-75%. Laparotomy by a skilled surgeon using intra-operative ultrasonography can give 80% or more accuracy of localisation. Surgical resection of the tumour in the pancreas is an alternative, but if unsuccessful or impracticable diazoxide, streptozotocin and somatostatin may be useful. It is also important to

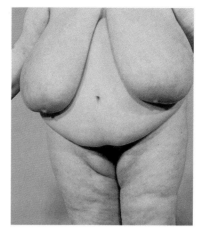

193

193 Insulinoma. Such overt obesity is sometimes a feature of insulinoma, although most with a weight problem are only modestly overweight.

remember that 10% of insulinoma patients may have multiple endocrine adenomatosis type 1 with associated hyperparathyroidism and pituitary tumours.

Nesidioblastoma is another rare condition, seen mainly in infants, where nesidioblasts differentiate from pancreatic duct epithelium and form A, B, D and pancreatic polypeptide cells which are separate from the true islets and increase the endocrine content of the pancreas five-fold. The picture is of a baby with somnolence, ataxia, fits and coma, often with brain damage due to hypoglycaemia. Treatment is by frequent feeds and diazoxide with pancreatectomy. Children with **Beckwith-Wiedemann syndrome** are characterised by gigantism, visceromegaly, mild microcephaly, large tongues, omphalocele and mild obesity. There is diffuse enlargement of the adrenal fetal cortex and hyperplasia of the kidneys, pancreas and gonadal interstitial cells. Although not a constant finding, hypoglycaemia of varying severity and duration has been reported in many of these infants.

There are many other causes of hypoglycaemia due to inborn errors of enzymatic metabolism. Recently, such errors have been detected in adults, (e.g. glycogen storage disease) some of whom develop weight gain and even mild obesity owing to their need to take frequent carbohydrate meals.

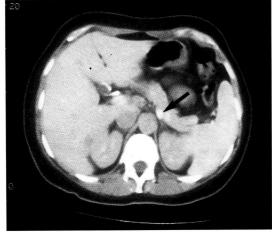

194 Insulinoma CAT scan. Following intravenous contrast a densely enhancing lesion can be seen in the body of the pancreas (arrowed) (ref. 26).

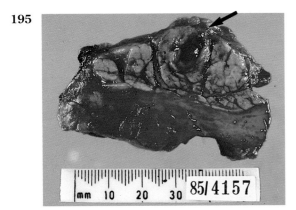

195 Insulinoma. Note the circumscribed, rounded lesion in the centre of the pancreas (arrowed)(ref. 26).

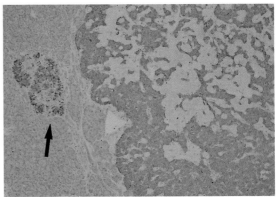

196 Insulinoma histology. Stained by immunoperoxidase which colours cells containing insulin dark brown. The area of deeper brown staining on the right is the insulinoma. On the left normal pancreas is seen with a single normal islet (arrow) (ref. 26).

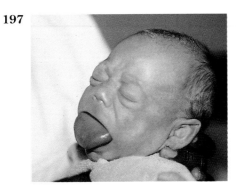

197 Beckwith-Weidemann syndrome is characterised by a large tongue.

198 Beckwith-Weidemann syndrome. This child was slightly taller than his peers and had mild obesity.

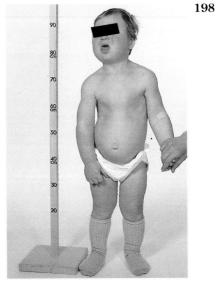

Hyperlipidaemia

Lipid Physiology

Cholesterol from the diet is incorporated at the intestinal level into chylomicrons which then pass into the blood circulation via the intestinal lymphatics. Chylomicrons vary in size from 80 to 500 nm and consist of a core of triglyceride and cholesterol esters surrounded by a coat of phospholipids, free cholesterol and apoproteins. The enzyme, lipoprotein lipase, found on vascular, endothelial cell walls, removes triglyceride from the chylomicrons in the peripheral circulation, forming a partially triglyceride-depleted chylomicron remnant which is then taken up by the liver. The liver secretes very low density lipoprotein (VLDL), consisting of endogenously synthesised triglyceride, and also cholesterol, which is both of endogenous and dietary (from the absorbed chylomicrons) origin. Once again the vascular endothelial lipoprotein lipase removes triglycerides from VLDL yielding fatty acids which are utilised by the tissues. As triglyceride is removed from the VLDL the particle shrinks, becoming denser, forming an intermediate density lipoprotein (IDL), which is either taken up by the liver or remains in the peripheral circulation, being further depleted of triglyceride to form a low density lipoprotein (LDL). About one half of LDL is then taken up by the liver and the rest by peripheral cells. As LDL is the major carrier of cholesterol in the plasma, this process of peripheral cell uptake is the major source of cholesterol for most tissues since only the liver, small intestine and skin have substantial rates of local cholesterol synthesis. (see **199**)

The uptake of LDL is efficient owing to high affinity receptors whose number is regulated by the cells' cholesterol content. The receptor recognises apoproteins B100 and E in the LDL particle. Any abnormality of these apoproteins results in a build up of LDL in the plasma. Should this occur the LDL can be taken up by unregulated processes, resulting in foam cells as seen in xanthoma and in atheromatous plaques. The liver cells also have the ability to synthesise cholesterol from acetyl coenzyme A by the rate-limiting enzyme, hydroxymethyl glutaryl coenzyme A (HMGCoA) reductase. Bile salts are synthesised from the pool of cholesterol in the liver cells.

High density lipoproteins (HDL) are a heterogenous group of particles which carry 20-30% of the total plasma-cholesterol. The liver secretes these lipid-poor particles of apoprotein and phospholipid which then accept cholesterol from cells. The cholesterol is then esterified by the enzyme, lecithin-cholesterol acyl transferase (LCAT), contained within the HDL particle. Hence HDL is involved in reverse cholesterol transport as free cholesterol is accepted, esterified and transferred to other lipoproteins, such as VLDL, and eventually to the liver. The protective effect of HDL against atheroma is derived from its ability to transport cholesterol from peripheral cells to the liver. IDL and LDL, on the other hand, deliver cholesterol to the arterial wall and hence are highly atherogenic. High levels of chylomicrons are not atherogenic but can cause pancreatitis.

Causes of Hyperlipidaemia

Primary

The primary hyperlipidaemic states are classified from I to V (Frederickson) in terms of the abnormal lipoprotein levels present. Some states are definitely associated with obesity, for example type IV and V, whereas other occur predominantly in the non-obese but weight excess exaggerates the problem. The Frederickson classification can describe a lipoprotein picture due to a single disorder, for example in type III in which there is a genetic abnormality of ApoE, but more often a specific type has more than one cause. There are a number of specific, inherited disorders of lipid metabolism which cause marked hyperlipidaemia (e.g. homozygous familial hypercholesterolaemia), but the majority of subjects have modest elevation of lipid levels owing to the effects of diet upon a predisposition by polygenic inheritance. This is often termed 'common polygenic hypercholesterolaemia' (type HA) and is associated with an increased risk of coronary heart disease, a tendency to develop corneal arcus and xanthelasma but not xanthomata. This type is found not only in the non-obese but can be seen in the obese where their weight (or intake) exacerbates the problem. There is an analogous situation as regards raised triglyceride levels. In 'common polygenic hypertriglyceridaemia' (type IV) VLDL levels are raised but HDL cholesterol is low. However, obesity is seen in over 90% of subjects with type IV hyperlipidaemia.

Table 23. Classification of Primary Hyperlipidaemias

Type (Frederickson)	Lipoprotein	Cause
I	Chylomicron increased HDL, LDL reduced	Lipoprotein lipase deficiency ApoC II deficiency
IIA	LDL increased Common polygenic hypercholesterolaemia Multiple type hyperlipidaemia	Familial hypercholesterolaemia
IIB	LDL, VLDL increased HDL reduced	Multiple type hyperlipidaemia Familial hypercholesterolaemia
III	IDL, chylomicrons remants increased LDL, HDL reduced	Abnormality of ApoE
IV*	VLDL increased HDL reduced Familial hypertriglyceridaemia Multiple type hyperlipidaemia	Common polygenic hypertriglyceridaemia
V*	VLDL, chylomicrons increased HDL, LDL reduced Lipoprotein lipase deficiency	Multiple type hyperlipidaemia Familial hypertriglyceridaemia

*Particularly associated with obesity

The familial hypercholesterolaemias are classified in two groups (type IIa and IIb) and represent autosomal, dominantly inherited disorders characterised by hypercholesterolaemia present from birth. The heterozygous form is said to affect 1 in 500 subjects, but a severe homozygous form can occur. The metabolic defect is an impaired (heterozygous) or absent (homozygous) high affinity pathway for LDL cholesterol catabolism. The disease manifests with both tendon and sheet xanthomata, corneal arcus and xanthelasma in childhood. Type III hyperlipidaemia is associated with cutaneous xanthomata, often taking the form of tuberous swellings over the elbows and elsewhere, with fatty streaks in the creases of the palms.

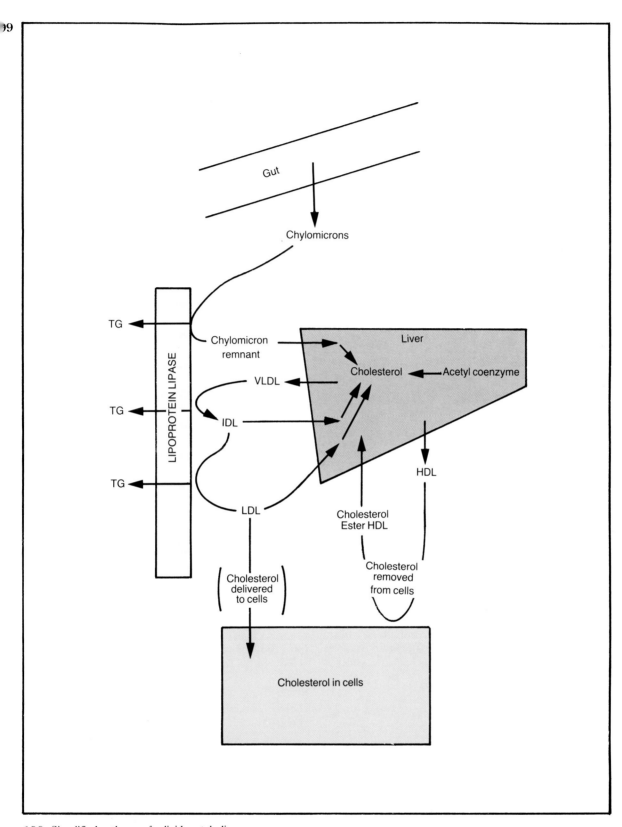

199 Simplified pathways for lipid metabolism.

There are two further types, namely, type I and V hyperlipidaemia. Type I is an autosomal, recessive condition which is usually present from birth and often manifests with relapsing pancreatitis. Eruptive xanthomata on back, buttocks, knees and elbows, retinal lipaemia, hepatosplenomegaly and chylomicronaemia are seen. Type V is clinically similar to type I except it is of dominant transmission and presentation most commonly occurs in adult life. Many are obese with glucose intolerance.

Hypertriglyceridaemia is consistently present, cholesterol levels raised and HDL cholesterol low. Eruptive xanthomata, pancreatitis and hepatosplenomegaly are often found.

There is also a 'multiple type hyperlipidaemia' in which the lipoprotein pattern varies in the affected members of a given family with types IIa, IIb, IV and V occurring. In this the hyperlipidaemia is seldom severe and so xanthomata are usually not observed.

Secondary

Causes of secondary hyperlipidaemia are:

- Dietary
- Diabetes
- Obesity
- Hypothyroidism
- Chronic renal failure
- Nephrotic syndrome
- Dysglobulinaemia
- Alcohol
- Drugs e.g. oral contraceptives
            thiazide diuretics
            beta blockers

Treatment

Emphasis should be on the diet. This should:

a) reduce total fat intake by stages so that fat makes up only 20% of the daily energy intake

b) substitute polyunsaturates, for example, by using olive, soya, corn, safflower or sunflower cooking oils. Some vegetable oils such as palm and coconut oils used in milk substitutes are saturated and should be avoided

c) reduce cholesterol rich foods such as liver, offal, egg yolks, fish roes and crustaceans (e.g. prawns). Aim for 100-150 mg cholesterol per day.

d) increase fibre

e) reduce weight in obese

f) reduce alcohol consumption

If, after three months of dietary compliance serum cholesterol triglyceride levels are elevated, other drugs such as bezafibrate, gemfibrozil or nicotinic acid (or analogues) may be required. A raised triglyceride alone may be reduced using omega-3, long chain fatty acids derived from fish oils. If cholesterol alone is markedly elevated then bile salt-binding resins such as cholestyramine, colestipol and probucol may be required.

A new development is the introduction of specific inhibitors of the rate-limiting enzyme of cholesterol synthesis, HMGCoA reductase, which can lower LDL cholesterol by up to 45%.

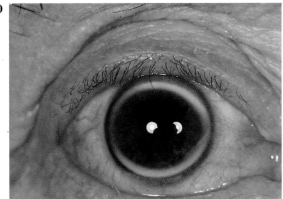

200 Arcus senilis in a patient with type IIA familial hypercholesterolaemia. This feature especially indicates hyperlipidaemia if found in the younger patient.

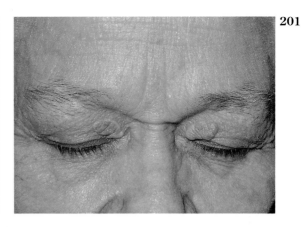

201 Xanthelasma involving the medial aspects of the upper eyelids.

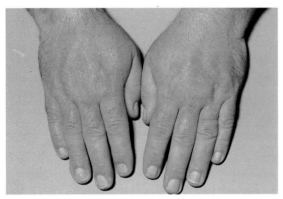

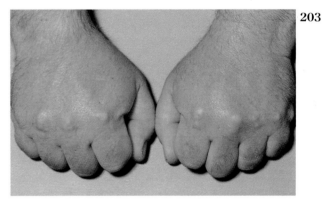

202 & 203 Tendon xanthomata may not be initially apparent (**202**) until the hand is flexed (**203**) when they are obvious over the knuckles.

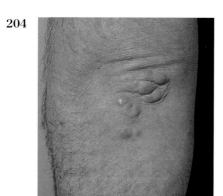

204 Xanthomata over the elbow.

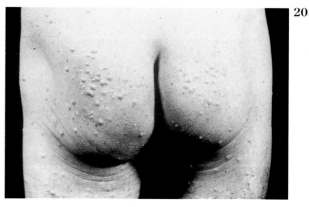

205 Eruptive xanthomata over the buttocks.

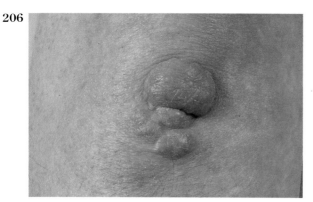

206 Tuberous xanthomata over the elbows.

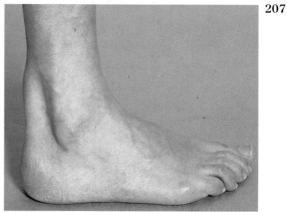

207 Thickening of achilles tendon due to hyperlipidaemia deposits.

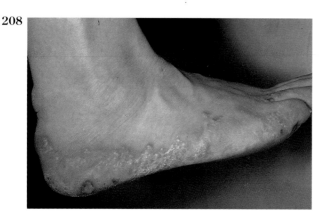

208 Achilles tendon thickening in this patient was associated with small, scattered xanthomata over the sole of the foot.

Abnormal fat distribution

The lipodystrophies comprise a group of disorders in which there is either abnormal fat distribution or the adipose mass is atrophic.

Generalised lipoatrophy (congenital generalised lipodystrophy) is exceptionally rare and is characterised by loss of adipose tissue throughout the body. This disorder may be congenital or acquired, with females involved more often than males. The clinical features associated with this form include acanthosis nigricans, splenomegaly, hyperlipidaemia, hyperglycaemia, marked insulin resistance, hypermetabolism, renal disease, cirrhosis, hirsutism, polycystic ovarian syndrome and generalised hyperpigmentation.

Partial lipoatrophy (lipodystrophy progressiva) is a more common disorder. Symmetrical loss of subcutaneous fat occurs over dermatome areas of the face and upper body, associated with normal or even excessive amounts of adipose tissue below the waist. Sometimes the atrophy involves the adipose tissue below the waist without involving the upper body. Almost all the clinical and biochemical abnormalities described for the generalised disorder have been reported in subjects with the partial form. Hyperlipidaemia associated with lipoatrophy is usually of the type IV or V variety and triglyceride elevations can be marked.

209

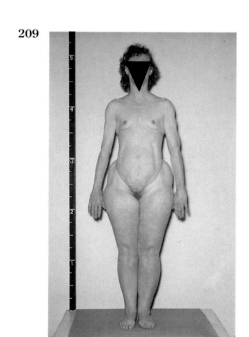

209 Partial lipoatrophy. Symmetrical loss of subcutaneous fat over the upper body associated with excessive fat deposition over the hips, thighs and lower legs.

Lipomatosis and Dercum's disease

Lipomas are benign mesenchymal tumours of adipose tissue. Most commonly they occur in the subcutaneous tissue but can be found in the retroperitoneum, mediastinum and elsewhere. In most cases they are of no consequence and require no therapy.

Dercum's disease (adiposis dolorosa) is a rare, progressive disease characterised by painful, subcutaneous fatty plaques often symmetrically localised to the lower extremities. It most commonly affects menopausal women who are usually obese at the onset of the disorder. Some families show a dominant inheritance. Histopathology reveals a combination of fat cell necrosis and interstitial tissue proliferation. Loss of weight and asthenia occurs as the disease progresses and juxta articular lesions may produce joint pains. Other commonly associated symptoms include severe emotional disturbance, amenorrhoea and sparseness of pubic and axillary hair. Intravenous lidocaine or mexilitene may be helpful.

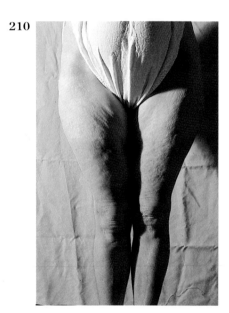

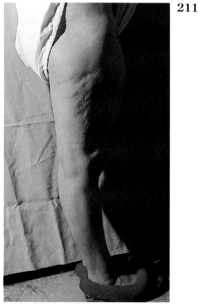

210 Dercum's disease. Painful, subcutaneous, fatty plaques symmetrically localised over the thighs.

211 Dercum's disease. The characteristic surface sensation on palpation is that of a 'bag of worms', also visible on this lateral thigh photograph.

6 Cardiovascular and Lymphatic Abnormalities

Table 24. Mortality Risk		
	Males	Females
Diabetes Mellitus	5.19	7.90
Digestive Diseases	3.99	2.29
Coronary Heart Disease	1.85	2.07
Cerebral Vascular Disease	2.27	1.52
Cancer (all sites)	1.33	1.55
		(ref.27)

Table 24 shows the mortality risk in those weighing 140% or more above an average weight (100%). This is compared to those 90-109% of average weight (1.0).

212 Mortality in obese males. In a recent analysis of 750,000 men and women in the USA the mortality rates for weights 120-129%, 130-139% and 140% or above were respectively 28%, 46% and 88% higher than for those of average weight (ref. 27). Although smoking is associated with a lower body weight, the mortality risk associated with smoking is far greater than that incurred by a modest weight gain. The mortality risk of smoking 20 cigarettes per day for a normal weight individual is similar to the mortality risk of being 140% above ideal weight. Females show a somewhat similar pattern (ref. 1).

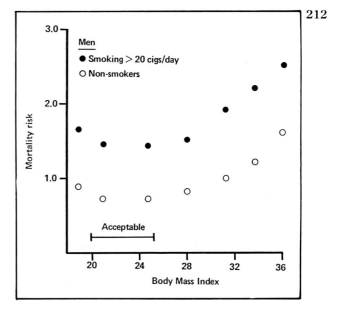

Table 25. Morbidity in obesity

Cardiovascular	Hypertension Coronary artery disease Cerebrovascular disease Peripheral vascular disease Varicose veins Varicose ulcers Ankle swelling Deep venous thrombosis Pulmonary embolism	Neurology	Nerve entrapment (e.g. neuralgia paraesthetica)
		Renal	Proteinuria
		Breast	Gynaecomastia in males Breast cancer
		Uterus	Endometrial cancer Cervical cancer
Respiratory	Breathless Pickwickian syndrome Cor pulmonale Sleep apnoea	Urological	Prostate cancer
		Skin	Sweat rashes Fungal infections Striae Lymphoedema Dry ulcers Cellulitis
Gastrointestinal	Hiatus hernia Gallstones and cholelithiasis Gallbladder and biliary cancers Fatty liver Constipation Haemorrhoids Herniae Cancer of colon and rectum	Operations	Respiratory risk Poor wound healing Ventral herniae Post-operative infections
Metabolic	Hyperlipidaemia Diabetes mellitus Polycystic ovarian syndrome Acanthosis nigricans Hirsutism Menstrual irregularities and menorrhagia	Orthopaedic	Spinal disc problems Osteoarthritis Exacerbates effect of all arthritides Gout Baker's cyst rupture
		Psychological disturbances **Pregnancy**	

Table 26. Morbidity risk for very obese women aged 30-49 years

Diabetes mellitus	4.5 x
Hypertension	3.3 x
Cholelithiasis	2.7 x
Gout	2.6 x
Arthritis (all causes)	1.6 x
Heart disease	1.6 x
Jaundice (all causes)	1.4 x

Coronary Heart Disease

Obesity is usually considered to be a less important risk factor than age, sex, blood pressure, smoking and hyperlipidaemia. Cigarette smoking is the greatest risk factor in younger men, whereas blood pressure is relatively more important in older age groups. Relative weight appears to be a direct risk factor only below the age of 50 years in males.

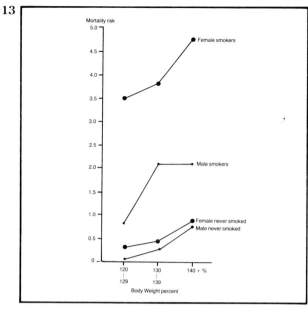

213 Mortality risk from coronary heart disease in males and females according to whether they smoke more than 20 cigarettes per day or whether they have never smoked. Note that the risk rises with weight in all groups (ref. 27).

214 Exercise treadmill test to detect ischaemic heart disease. Leads attached to the patient's chest detect electrocardiographic changes monitored on the oscilloscope.

215 Positive exercise test with ST depression in the chest leads V4 and V5 after eight minutes of exercise.

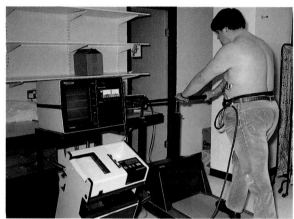

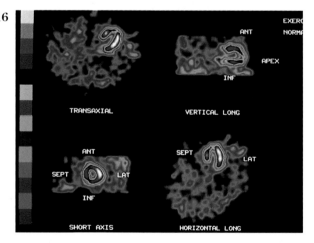

216 Thallium scan. A normal scan during exercise.

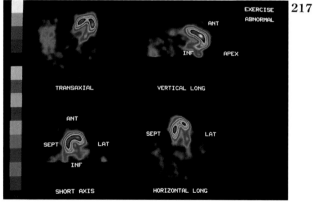

217 Ischaemic thallium scan. With exercise this patient showed inferolateral ischaemia. Note the lack of uptake of thallium in the appropriate inferior lateral segments.

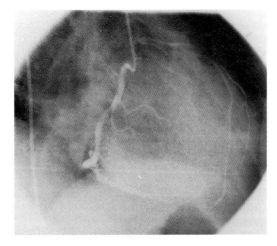

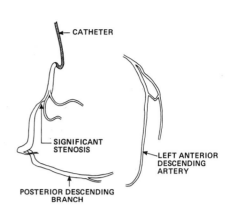

218 Coronary angiogram showing significant stenosis in the right coronary artery with the left anterior descending artery filling by collaterals.

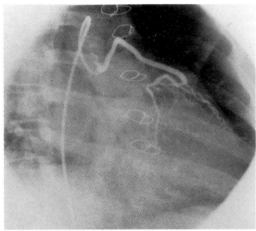

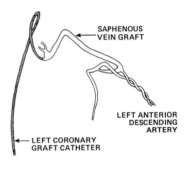

219 Coronary angiogram after saphenous vein graft relieved the patient of angina.

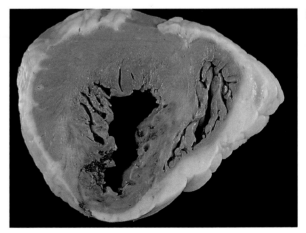

220 Fatty heart section through epicardium and myocardium revealing extensive fatty infiltration shown up in the lower picture as a red stain by Sudan IV.

221 Fatty heart. Transverse section through right and left ventricles shows extensive fat in the epicardium and a myocardial infarction involving the septum and left ventricle.

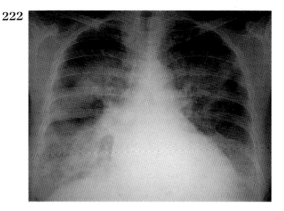

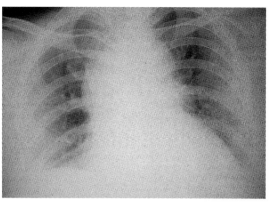

222 Pulmonary oedema due to a myocardial infarction showing characteristic congestion spreading out from the hilum.

223 Dissection of the aorta. Note the widened mediastinum due to splitting of the arch of the aorta. This patient also had aortic regurgitation because the dissection widened the aortic ring.

Hypertension and Cerebrovascular Disease

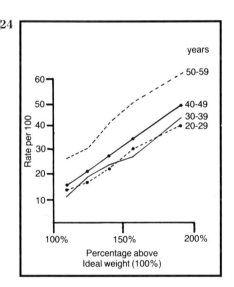

224

224 Hypertensive rate in obese women. The older and heavier the woman, the greater the risk of hypertension. Similar results have been reported in males. Framingham data has shown that there is a 6 mm rise in systolic blood pressure and a 4 mm rise in diastolic blood pressure with a 10% gain in body fat (ref. 28).

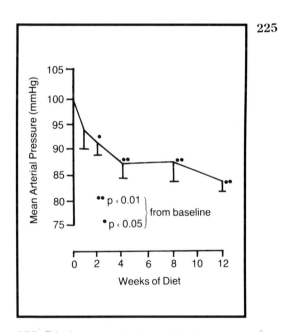

225

225 Dieting reduces blood pressure in hypertensive patients. Twenty-five obese patients on a 320 kcal (1.3 MJ/per day) slimming diet containing 110 mmol of sodium showed significant falls in mean arterial pressure. By the 12th week the average weight loss was 20.2 kg and the average fall in mean arterial pressure was 17 mmHg (ref. 29).

226 Cafe au lait patches in this hypertensive young women led to the eventual diagnosis of phaeochromocytoma. The right adrenal tumour was removed, resulting in the relief of her hypertension. Most patients with phaeochromocytoma are not obese but this case illustrates the need to think of the remedial causes of hypertension in the obese. Another example is shown in **216** where the patient illustrated has primary hyperaldosteronism as the cause of his hypertension.

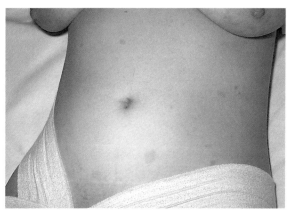

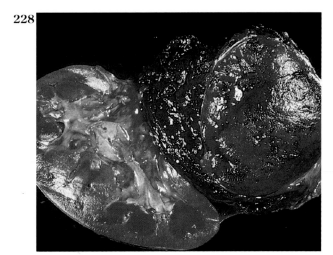

227 ^{131} **iodine-meta iodobenzylguanide (MIGB) scan.** This can sometimes be helpful in detecting a phaeochromocytoma (arrowed) and secondaries if present. The kidney is outlined with DMSA (picture on left).

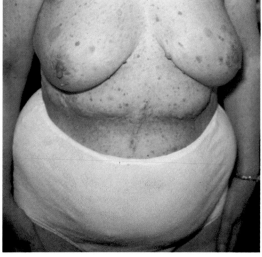

228 Phaeochromocytoma removed at operation. Kidney is shown on the left with a large phaeochromocytoma involving the adrenal with associated haemorrhage.

229 Neurofibromatosis. Phaeochromocytoma can be found in association with neurofibromatosis as well as multiple endocrine adenomatosis type II and type III, Von-Hippel-Lindau disease and tuberose sclerosis.

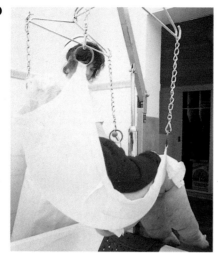

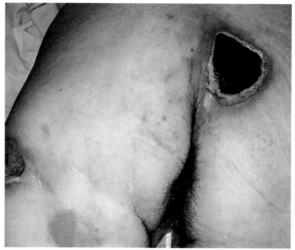

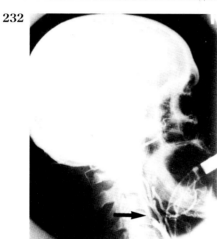

232

230 Cerebrovascular disease produced a stroke in this elderly, obese woman. Her obesity made physical aspects of nursing difficult. Bathing necessitated using a special harness and crane device.

231 Pressure sores. This patient was initially nursed at home where the pressure sores developed. Good nursing care to prevent this is vital in the obese.

232 Transient ischaemic attacks in this patient were due to internal carotid artery stenosis (arrow). This is amenable to surgical correction.

Cardiovascular Disease

233 Atheroma of aorta and iliac arteries. The patient had Leriche syndrome with ischaemic pain in the thigh and buttocks.

234 Small aneurysm of abdominal aorta gave rise to an abdominal bruit.

233 234

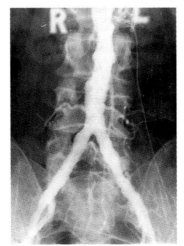

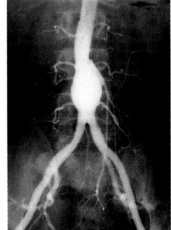

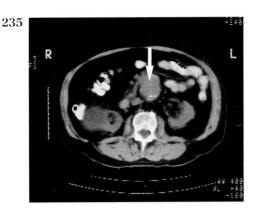
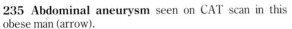

235 Abdominal aneurysm seen on CAT scan in this obese man (arrow).

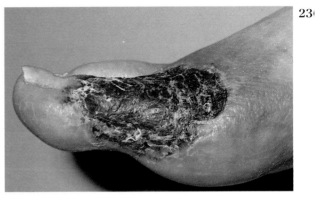

236 Necrotic arteriopathic ulcer in a severely ischaemic foot.

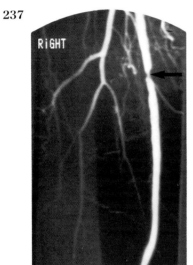

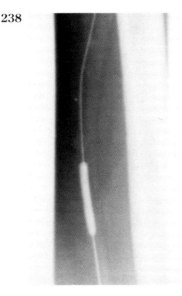

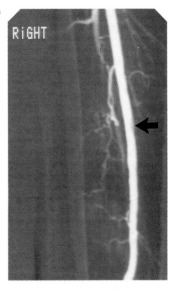

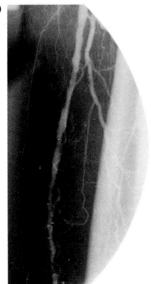

237 Atheromatous stenosis of femoral artery (arrow) resulted in severe intermittent claudication. Such a lesion is amenable to angioplasty.

238 Angioplasty balloon which was threaded down the femoral artery and the balloon expanded to open up the stenosis.

239 Relieved stenosis (shown by arrow) by angioplasty of patient in **237**.

240 Severe atheroma in femoral artery is not usually amenable to angioplasty and often requires open surgery.

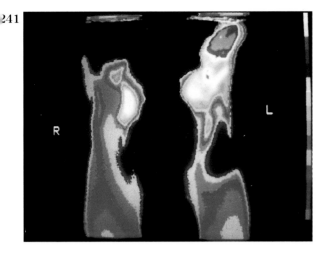

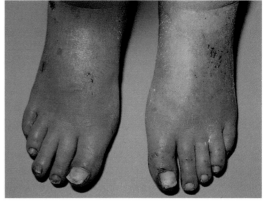

241 **Thermal imaging** shows a right ischaemic foot.

242 **Frost bite** in an obese woman.

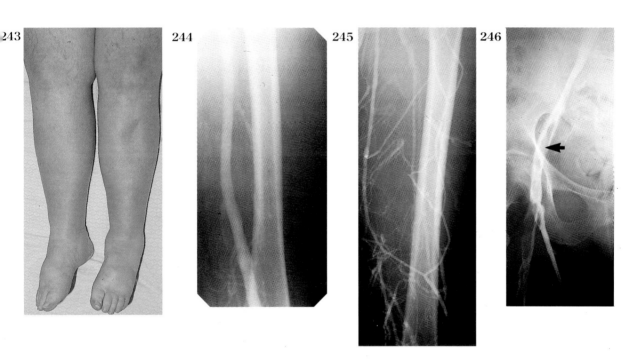

243 **Deep venous thrombosis** is more common in obese subjects, especially after operations and in women after pregnancy. Recurrent bilateral problem in this patient.

244 **Normal femoral vein.**

245 **Thrombosis of femoral vein** has resulted in the opening of collateral vessels.

246 **Thrombus** in iliac vein lying loose in the lumen (arrow). This can be dangerous as the clot may become dislodged and cause pulmonary embolism.

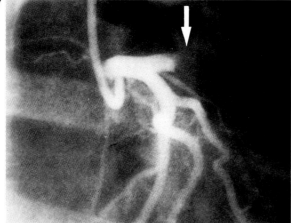

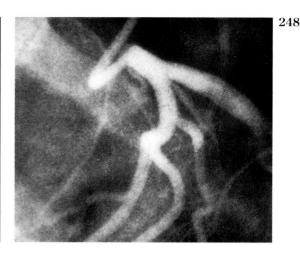

247 Pulmonary embolism showing the embolus blocking one of the main arterial channels (arrow).

248 Streptokinase was infused thrombolysing the clot which had blocked the branch of the pulmonary artery shown in **247**.

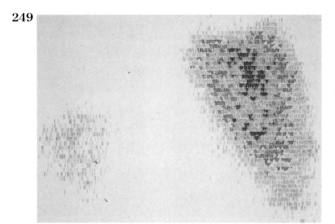

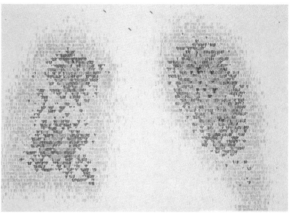

249 Perfusion lung scan showing a lack of perfusion to the upper part of the right lung due to a massive pulmonary embolism.

250 Perfusion lung scan after streptokinase had removed the clot and allowed some reperfusion to the upper lung on the right side.

251 Phlegmasia coerulia dolens is a rare but severe form of deep venous thrombosis due to occlusion of all the main venous drainage of a limb. Note the oedema with tense serous bullae, deroofed bullae and gangrene of the toes of the left foot. The oedema is thought to cause arterial occlusion coupled with intravascular volume depletion, resulting in peripheral ischaemia and eventual gangrene (ref. 30).

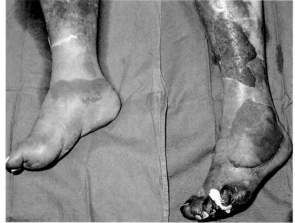

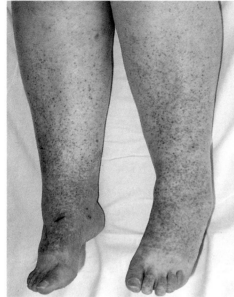

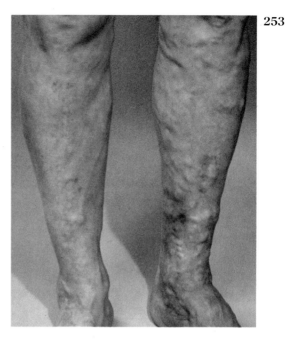

252 Purpura on this obese woman's legs was due to idiopathic thrombocytopenic purpura.

253 Varicose veins. A common cause is deep venous thrombosis which causes valvular incompetence of the perforating vessels between the deep and superficial leg veins. Hence, venous blood under high pressure is forced from the deep to the superficial vessels causing massive dilatation as shown. Obese women, who have several children, are often prone to varicose veins possibly due to post-thrombotic state after childbirth.

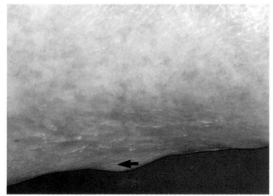

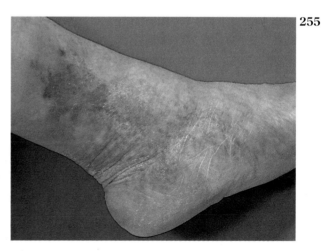

254 An incompetent perforating vessel allowing blood to leak from the deep to the superficial venous system (arrow).

255 Varicose eczema and pigmentation due to an incompetent perforating vessel. Raised capillary pressure forces red cells into the surrounding tissue where haemosiderosis stains the tissues. Eczema often begins in the area of pigmentation and such irritation can also increase pigmentation by melanin production.

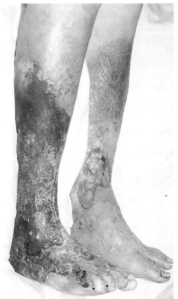

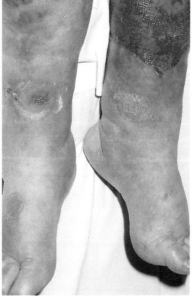

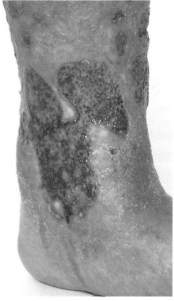

256 Severe pigmentation due to varicose stasis, eczema and infection.

257 Leg ulcer due to infected areas of varicose eczema in association with oedema.

258 Varicose ulcers can be extensive and indolent. Note the areas of healing skin leaving islands of ulceration.

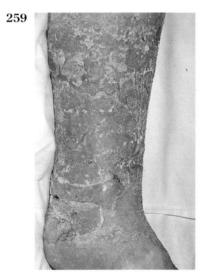

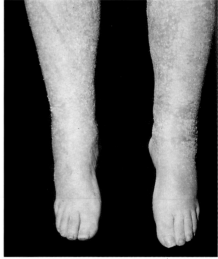

259 Stasis eczema can be extensive and an irritant. Sudden exacerbation of the eczematous area can result in a generalised eczematous eruption on face and forearms.

260 Asteototic eczema involving both legs.

Lymphoedema

The cause of lymph stasis can be inherited or acquired. In the **congenital type** (Milroy's disease), oedema of the lower limbs can present at birth (congenital lymphoedema), be delayed to childhood, adolescence or young adulthood (lymphoedema praecox), or occur after the age of 30 (lymphoedema tarda). In the early stages the oedema can be asymetrical but later both legs can become affected.

The swelling may cease at the ankle in the early stages and in some cases at the knee. Ultimately it reaches the groin above which it seldom extends, although scrotum, penis or vulva may also be involved. The cause is a congenital anomaly of the draining lymphatics of the lower limbs and lymphangiography demonstrates either aplasia, hypoplasia (most common) or varices of the lymph channels.

Acquired lymphoedema may be due to **trauma** such as after radical mastectomy for breast cancer, repeat lower limb cellulitic **infections**, chronic infections such as tuberculosis, filariasis and fungal infections, **operations for varicose veins** and obstruction by **malignant** diseases.

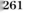

262

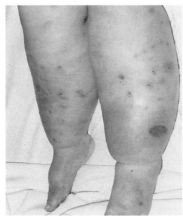

261

263

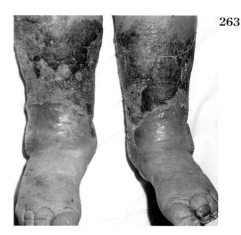

261 Bilateral lymphoedema with resultant ulceration. Lymphoedema mainly involves the subcutaneous tissues, where there is an increase in the stagnant lymphatic channels in supporting fat and fibrous tissue. Note the demarcation at the ankle.

262 Symmetrical lymphoedema. The skin becomes wrinkled, coarsened and folded with extensive, brown areas of dry, undesquamated keratin.

263 Ulceration on both lymphoedematous legs.

264

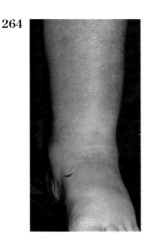

265

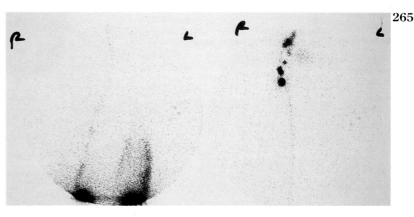

264 Cellulitis. Episodes often occur in a lymphoedematous leg. Each such attack makes the obstruction worse and the swelling thus increases.

265 Isotopic lymphangiogram of a swollen left leg. This patient had had repeated cellulitic episodes involving the left leg. The isotope was injected subcutaneously

between the toe webs in each foot as shown on the left isotopic picture. On the right isotopic picture isotope has reached the groin lymph nodes of the right leg but no uptake is seen over the left groin nodes. This confirmed congenital lymphoedema tarda of the left leg.

266
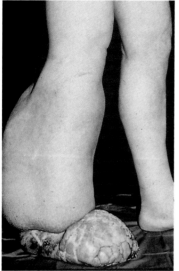

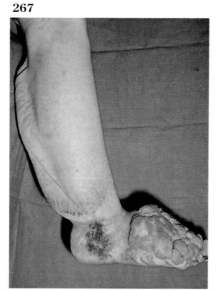

26
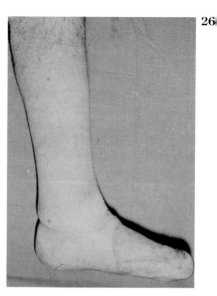

266 Gross lymphoedematous disfigurement can be improved by plastic surgery.

267 Compression operation. The leg is compressed for several days to relieve the oedema. The residual skin and subcutaneous tissue are removed and partial amputation with plastic repair is carried out on the foot.

268 End result of operation is an acceptable cosmetic effect.

269 Compression boot. Stockings and a supportive boot are used to try and prevent the leg swelling up again.

270 Ulcerated fat legs can occur in very obese individuals. Repeated infection in such an ulcer can eventually lead to acquired lymphoedema exacerbating the problem.

271 Fat ankles with cellulitis and ulcerations.

269
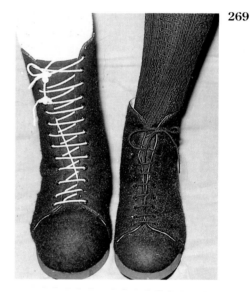

270
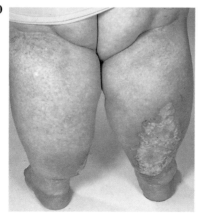

27
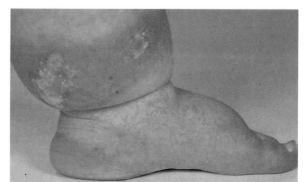

7 Cancer and Gastrointestinal Diseases

Table 27. Significant mortality risk of cancer in obese subjects.
Risk compared to those of 90-109% of average weight.

| Cancer | Weight Index | | |
	120-129%	130-139%	140 +%
Males			
Colon and rectum	NS	1.53	1.73
Prostate	1.37	1.33	1.29
Females			
Gallbladder and biliary passages	1.74	1.80	3.58
Endometrium	1.85	2.30	5.42
Cervix	1.51	1.42	2.39
Breast	NS	NS	1.53
Ovary	NS	NS	1.63
		(ref. 27)	

In an analysis of mortality by weight among 750,000 men and women in the USA, cancer mortality was increased, especially in those weighing 140% or more, with the risk being 1.33 and 1.55 times as great in males and females respectively as those weighing 90-109% of average weight (ref. 27). As **Table 27** shows, colorectal cancer was the principal site of excess cancer mortality in males (1.73 in males, 1.22 in females). In females the highest incidence was for endometrial cancer (5.42), followed by cancer of the gallbladder and biliary passage (3.58), which are uncommon cancers. In addition, with increasing weight, there appears to be a progressive increase in cancer risk for the cervix, breast and ovary. Mortality risk from digestive diseases also increases with weight, more so in males than females. Gallbladder disease is the most common form of digestive disease in obese individuals. This is seen particularly in Pima Indians where the prevalence in women aged 15-24 years is 13%, rising to 73% in the 25-34 years group (ref. 31). Among Pima men the prevalence at 25-34 years is 4%, rising to 68% in those over 65 years of age. Rimm and colleagues, in a study of over 70,000 obese women in the USA and Canada, reported a 2.7-fold increase in the prevalence of gallbaldder disease (ref. 28). In the Framingham study the incidence is twice as high in women as in men, increases with age and weight in both sexes and rises with the number of pregnancies (ref. 32). Weight and age appear additive but it appears that obesity is six times more important than age.

The mechanism for all this appears to be due to the excretion of excessive amounts of cholesterol in bile. Bile is rendered soluble by bile salts but if the ratio of cholesterol to bile salts exceeds the saturation index then cholesterol precipitates out, forming gallstones. With advancing obesity, endogenous cholesterol synthesis by the liver and other tissues increases, eventually exceeding the saturation index. The predominance of gallbladder disease in women probably reflects the effect of natural oestrogen and exogenous oestrogen in the contraceptive pill on biliary cholesterol secretion and saturation. During slimming, cholesterol is mobilised from adipose tissue and the saturation index falls. Fibre appears to play an important role in a slimming diet for, if lacking, a reduced bile salt pool results, decreasing the solubilisation of excreted cholesterol and hence increasing the tendency to gallstone formation.

This lack of fibre in slimming diets may account for the increased incidence of constipation and diverticular disease in obese subjects.

Table 28. Digestive diseases. Mortality risk as compared to those 90-109% of average weight

Weight index	Males	Females
120-129	1.88	1.61
130-139	2.89	2.19
140 +	3.99	2.29
		(ref. 27)

272

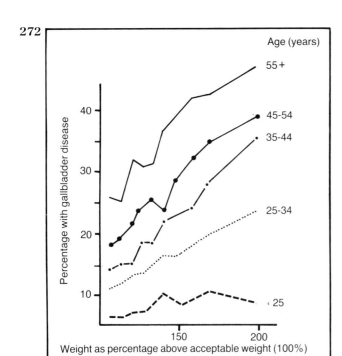

272 Relationship of gallbladder disease to weight and age in adult women in the USA. Note the rising incidence with age and obesity (ref. 34).

273

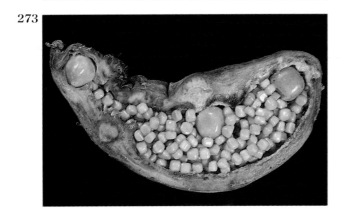

273 Gallstones in gallbladder. Note the abscesses in the thickened wall of the gallbladder.

274

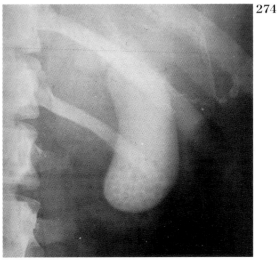

274 Multiple gallstones in a gallbladder visualised by contrast during oral cholecystography.

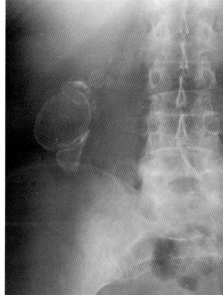

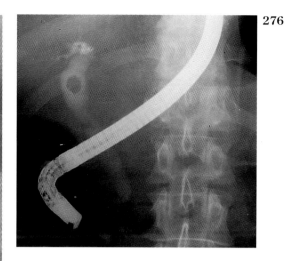

275 Massive calcified gallstones seen on plain abdominal X-ray.

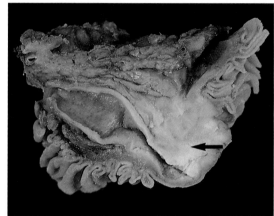

276 Gallstone in common bile duct caused repeated biliary colic and cholangitis. The stone was visualised using ERCP. A sphincterotomy done at ERCP released the stone.

277 Bile duct carcinoma (arrow) producing dilatation of the common bile duct.

278 Cancer of descending colon caused marked narrowing of the bowel (arrow).

279 Caecal carcinoma with typical apple-core picture (arrow).

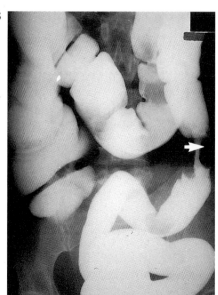

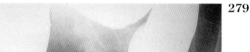
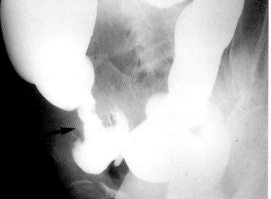

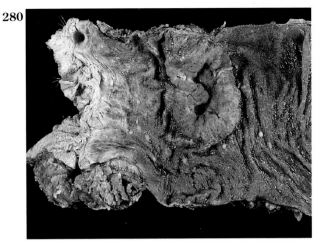

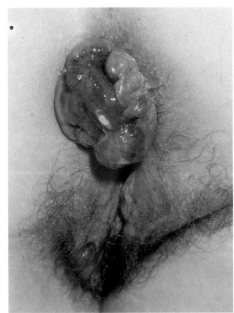

280 Rectal carcinoma. This cancer is seen as an unpigmented, rolled-edged ulcer. The pigmental rectal mucosa (melanosis coli) is due to laxative abuse. Note the multiple, unpigmented, metaplastic polyps.

281 Haemorrhoids are a problem in obesity possibly related to constipation, a consequence of low fibre slimming diets.

282 Diverticular disease with outpouchings from the sigmoid colon, again related to lack of dietary fibre and constipation.

283 Fatty liver. Unstained section showing the pale, amorphous nature of this fatty liver.

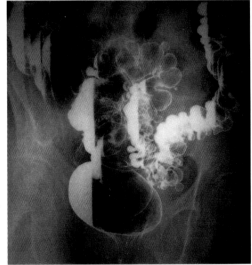

284 Fatty liver. Section of liver in **283**, stained for fat with Sudan Red, showing the extensive fat infiltration.

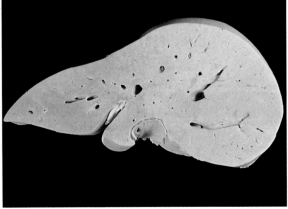

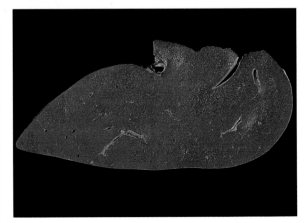

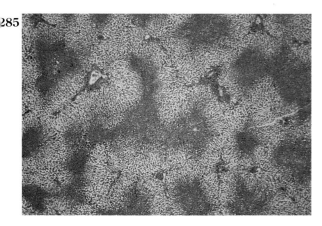

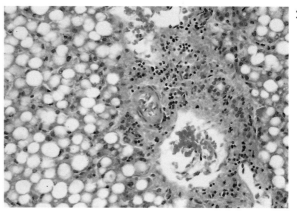

28

285 Fatty liver. Low-powered view showing fatty infiltration as shown by the paler areas.

286 Fatty liver. High-powered view of **285** showing globules of fat.

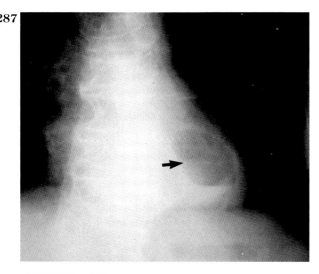

287 Hiatus hernia was observed on straight radiological view, as the stomach gas shadow (arrow) was seen overriding the left side of the heart.

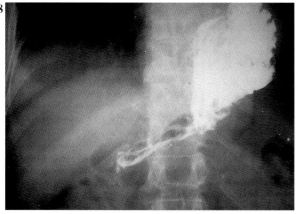

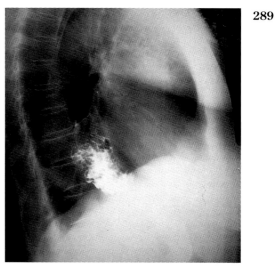

288 & 289 Hiatus hernia of **287** was confirmed by barium swallow — both on anteroposterior (**288**) and lateral views (**289**).

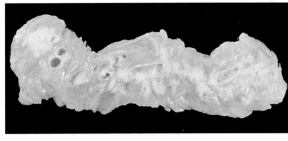

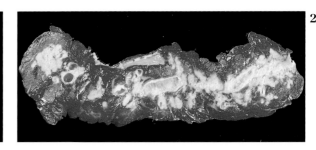

290 Pancreas heavily infiltrated with fat (unstained).

291 Fatty pancreas. Section of pancreas in **290**, stained for fat with Sudan Red, clearly showing the extensive fat deposition.

292

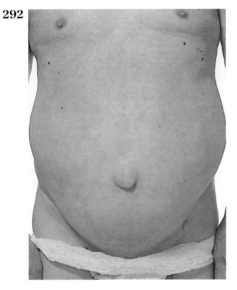

293

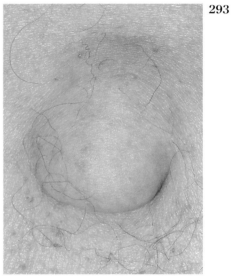

292 Umbilical hernia in a man with marked abdominal obesity.

293 Umbilical hernia close up view (from patient in **292**).

294

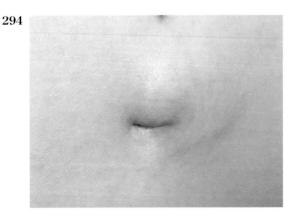

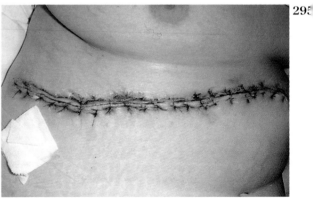

294 Sister Joseph's nodule. This is a metastatic tumour in the umbilicus from cancer of the colon. In this case the mass did not show a cough impulse and had a solid feel to it.

295 Incisional hernia repair. Incisional hernia can be a problem in the obese, in many cases associated with wound infection. Weight loss before repair often increases the chance that the repair will be successful and long-standing.

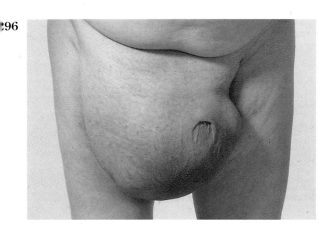

296 Hydrocele in an obese man with an extensive abdominal obesity.

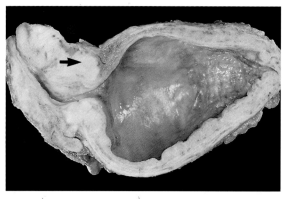

297 Prostatic carcinoma (arrow) with bladder.

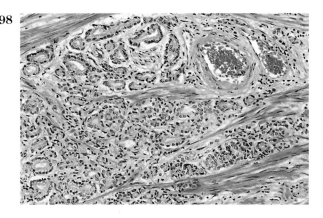

298 Prostatic carcinoma. High-powered view of **297** showing irregular acini and abnormal architecture.

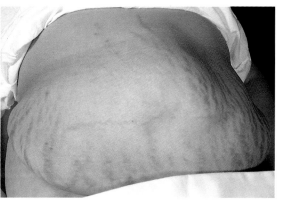

299 Incarcerated ventral hernia. To succeed operatively weight loss was imperative.

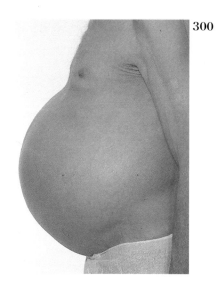

300 Ascites (and **not** abdominal obesity) due to excess alcohol intake. Alcohol excess often results in obesity which is frequently abdominal in distribution. This is accentuated if ascites develops.

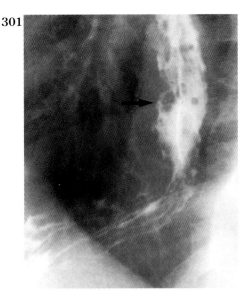

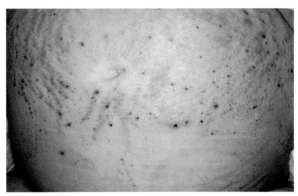

301 Oesophageal varices seen on this barium swallow (arrow) are a complication of alcoholic excess. Massive bleeding from varices is often fatal.

302 Cholestatic pruritus. Note the scratch marks and striae over this ascitic and obese abdomen.

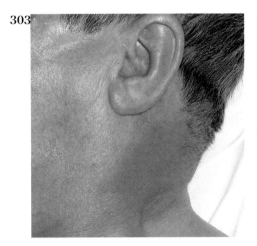

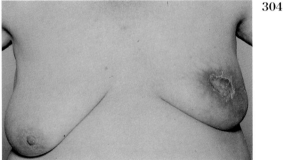

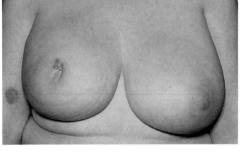

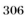

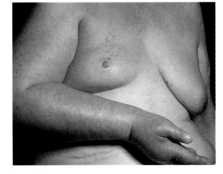

303 Alcoholic myalgia is due to necrosis of muscle brought about by alcoholic excess. The overlying skin becomes reddened and hot and the area is acutely tender (as seen behind his ear). This man also had an inflamed calf resembling a deep vein thrombosis. Myoglobin is released into the circulation and leads to renal failure, often fatal as in this case.

304 Breast cancer which has invaded the skin and partially ulcerated.

305 Breast cancer puckering and lifting the right nipple.

306 Breast cancer has advanced to include the lymph nodes draining the arm, resulting in lymphoedema of the arm.

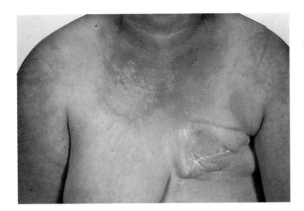

307 Dermatomyositis in a woman who previously had a breast cancer removed by mastectomy. Dermatomyositis can be precipitated by malignancy. It usually presents as an acute erythema of the light-exposed areas of the face and arms, associated with muscle weakness and wasting.

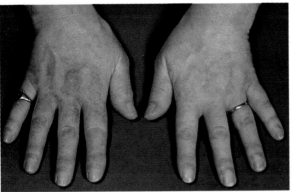

308 Dermatomyositis also produces a streaky erythema (Dowling's lines) over the tendons on the dorsum of the hands.

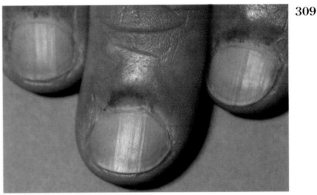

309 Telangectasia of nailbeds is also seen in dermatomyositis.

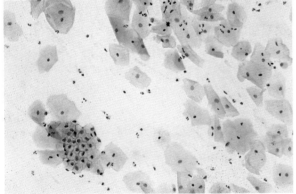

310 Normal cervical smear. This shows a clump of normal, honeycomb-like, endocervical cells with superficial and intermediate cells as well as scattered polymorphs.

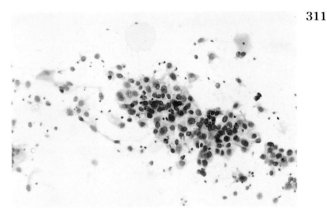

311 Dyskaryotic cervical smear. This would require a cone biopsy to exclude cancer.

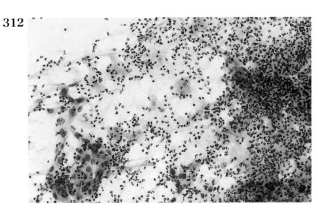

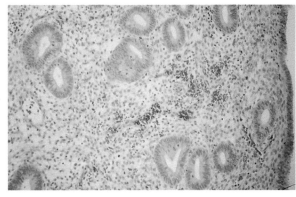

312 Squamous cell carcinoma in a cervical smear. Note the marked nuclear pleomorphism and prominent nucleoli with background tumour diathesis.

313 Normal endometrial tissue (ref. 33).

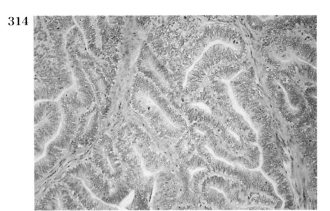

314 Well-differentiated endometrial cancer (ref. 33).

315 Ovarian tumour produced extensive abdominal distension and weight loss in this previously overweight woman. Note the femoral hernia.

316 Ovarian tumour removed from patient in **315** at operation.

317 Ovarian cyst produced extensive abdominal swelling in this overweight woman. Abdominal distension may not necessarily be solely due to obesity but can be due to enlarged bladder, ovarian pathology, ascites and even undiagnosed pregnancy.

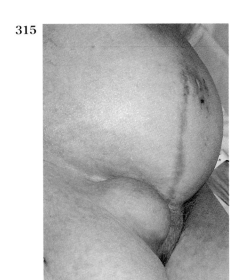

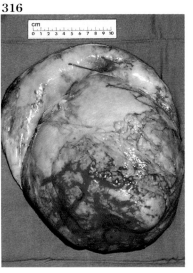

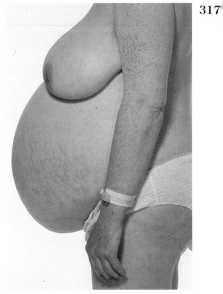

8 Insulin Resistance, Acanthosis Nigricans and Diabetes Mellitus

Insulin Resistance

In obesity there is hyperinsulinaemia and insulin resistance. Subjects with mild insulin resistance have a reduced number of insulin receptors, whereas those with a greater degree of insulin resistance exhibit both a reduction in insulin receptors and one or more post-receptor defects. In the severely insulin-resistant obese patient the post-receptor defects take prominence.

Acanthosis Nigricans

This skin condition is associated with variable degrees of insulin resistance. Initially the skin affected becomes dry and darkened and could be confused by the careless observer with an unwashed skin. Later, the dermis becomes thickened and may eventually become folded or warty in appearance. The lesions are often symmetrical and usually involve flexures such as the nape of the neck, axilla, infra-mammary folds, periareolar areas, groins and intergluteal cleft. Histological examination of these lesions shows increased keratin (hyperkeratosis) and epidermal hyperplasia (acanthosis) with upward projection of the dermal papillae (papillomatosis). Hyaluronic acid is found infiltrating the papillary dermis.

Despite confusing terminology, this skin condition does occur with different systemic associations. Firstly, it may be associated with various endocrine disorders such as acromegaly, gigantism, Addison's disease, Cushing's syndrome (especially if induced by exogenous steroids), lipoatrophic diabetes mellitus, partial lipodystrophy, leprechaunism and a rare form of severe insulin-resistant diabetes due to insulin receptor antibodies. The above need not be obese, indeed, except for Cushing's, most cases are of normal weight. The second association is with malignancy, especially gastrointestinal adenocarcinomas mainly of the stomach. This variety is usually seen in slim, middle-aged patients. It is usually severe and progresses rapidly in some, involving the whole skin. The pigmentation is also more prominent, hyperkeratosis of soles and palms may occur and, in half the patients, mucous membranes are involved, resulting in warty papillomatosis thickening around the lips. Onset of this form may precede evidence of a tumour by as much as five years and regression usually follows tumour removal.

The third form is not associated with malignancy but usually occurs with obesity. It is often inappropriately termed 'pseudoacanthosis nigricans' to distinguish this benign variety from the malignancy-associated type. This form mainly occurs in caucasian females with an onset at, or shortly after, puberty and is often associated with hirsutism and/or hyperandrogenaemia in females. It was previously thought to be a rare disorder but with increasing medical awareness the prevalence has risen. However, as yet, the actual figure is unknown with rates of 5-29% reported in patients referred to various specialist centres for evaluation of hirsutism and/or hyperandrogenaemia.

The most salient features include obesity, insulin resistance, occasionally with clinical manifestation of diabetes mellitus, gonadal dysfunction, mainly expressed in women as polycystic ovary syndrome, infertility, impotency, hirsutism, hyperandrogenaemia, virilism and in some auto-immune hypothyroidism. In males with this condition obesity, impotence, gonadal dysfunction and hypothyroidism have been reported.

In the obese with acanthosis nigricans, fasting insulin levels have been reported on average 15-fold higher than those found in matched, obese, non-acanthotic subjects, whose levels are 3-fold elevated compared to normal weight individuals. In contrast, non-acanthotic, obese women with hyperandrogenaemia have an average 5-fold increase in fasting insulin levels (ref. 35). In the same report the fall in plasma glucose to an intravenous insulin bolus was markedly impaired in those with acanthosis nigricans, being 30% of that seen in normal weight individuals, as compared with 78% of normal in matched obese and 40% of normal in hyperandrogenic women.

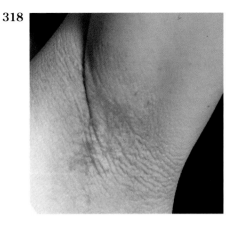

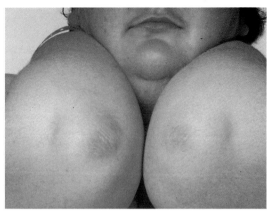

318 Acanthosis nigricans of the axilla showing the pigmented, thickened folds of skin associated with skin tags.

319 Acanthosis nigricans of the elbows in a patient with necrobiosis lipoidica. Note the symmetry of the skin lesion in that both elbows are involved (**319, 320, 321** and **322** are from the same patient).

Table 29. Response to 75 g glucose tolerance test				
	Acanthotic obese patient		Non-acanthotic obese females	
Time mins	Glucose mmol/l	Insulin u/l	Glucose mmol/l	Insulin u/l
0	4.8	36	4.9	19
30	8.5	121	8.1	94
60	11.2	186	8.0	101
90	10.0	203	6.7	75
120	8.2	206	6.4	66

Table 29 Insulin resistance occurs with acanthosis nigricans. 75 g glucose tolerance test is shown for the patient illustrated in **319-322**. Compared with the values obtained in 40 obese females of similar average weight.

The insulin resistance in acanthosis nigricans is generally associated with both receptor and post-receptor defects. There are, however, reports of a few obese patients having insulin receptor antibodies. This contrasts with the situation in thin individuals with acanthosis nigricans and diabetes mellitus where severe extremes of insulin resistance have been reported associated with a high prevalence of insulin receptor antibodies. In the obese acanthosis nigricans type, about one-fifth have overt clinical diabetes mellitus. The skin lesions appear to be due to the hyperinsulinaemia and not to the hyperandrogenaemia or to the obesity (see ref. 36, 37).

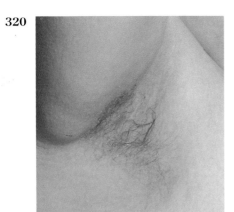

320 Axilla involved with acanthosis nigricans.

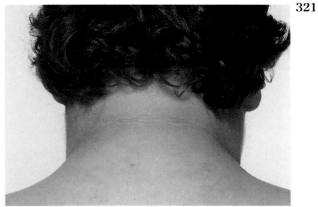

321 Acanthosis nigricans of nape of the neck.

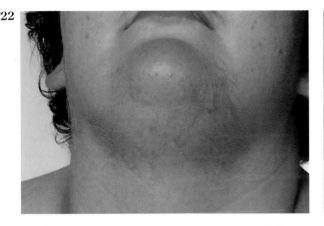

322 Mild hirsutism associated with acanthosis nigricans in this patient.

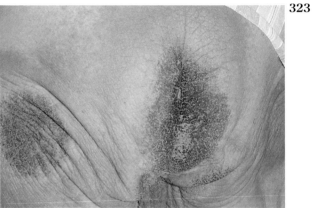

323 Intergluteal and buttock involvement with acanthosis nigricans.

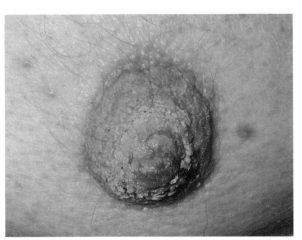

324 Acanthosis nigricans of the nipple and the areolar region.

325 Histology of acanthosis nigricans showing increased keratin, thickening of the epidermis and upward projection of the dermal papillae. Slight blue-purple haze is due to stained excess hyaluronic acid found infiltrating the dermis in this condition.

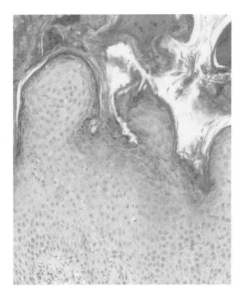

Diabetes Mellitus

The risk of developing maturity-onset diabetes increases with both the degree of obesity and the duration of obesity. This applies to both men and women. There is also an interaction between the familial tendency to maturity-onset diabetes and obesity. Data suggest that the incidence of diabetes mellitus among the children of a diabetic parent is more than doubled if the children are also obese. The risk of diabetes and other complications of obesity seems to be associated particularly with individuals with an android (abdominal) fat distribution.

326 Diabetes mellitus incidence increases both with the degree of obesity and with age as shown by the study of Rimm et al (1975) of 73,532 women (ref. 28).

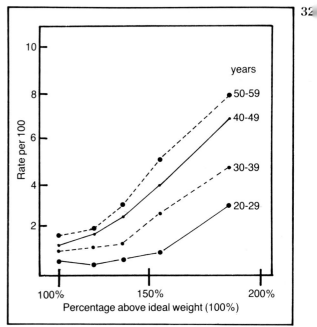

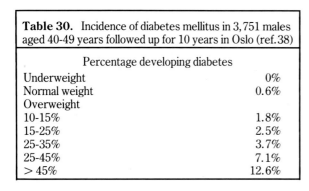

Table 30. Incidence of diabetes mellitus in 3,751 males aged 40-49 years followed up for 10 years in Oslo (ref.38)

Percentage developing diabetes	
Underweight	0%
Normal weight	0.6%
Overweight	
10-15%	1.8%
15-25%	2.5%
25-35%	3.7%
25-45%	7.1%
> 45%	12.6%

Table 31.	Complications of Diabetes Mellitus
Skin	— Stiff hand syndrome Necrobiosis lipoidica Dermopathy
Eye	— Maculopathy Retinopathy Vitreous haemorrhage Retinal detachment Rubeosis of iris Cataracts
Kidney	— Microalbuminuria Proteinuria Nephrotic syndrome Renal failure
Vascular	— Peripheral vascular disease Cerebrovascular disease Coronary artery disease Ischaemic ulcers
Neuropathy	— Polyneuropathy Mononeuritis Autonomic abnormalities Neuropathic ulceration Charcot joint
Infections	— Bacterial e.g. osteomyelitis Boils Fungal Tuberculosis
Impotence **Coma**	— Hypoglycaemia Ketoacidosis Hyperosmolar Lactic acidosis

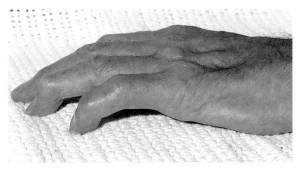

327 Stiff hand of a longstanding, diabetic patient showing wasting of the small muscles of the hand, especially the interossei, and restricted mobility of the joints with the fingers permanently flexed. The skin is thick, tight and waxy. This is the result of thickening of dermal collagen and is an early indicator of microvascular complications.

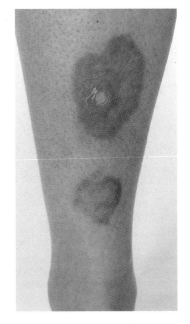
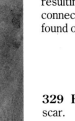

328 Necrobiosis lipoidica is due to small vessel damage resulting in partial necrosis of dermal collagen and connective tissue cells. More common in females and often found on the shins.

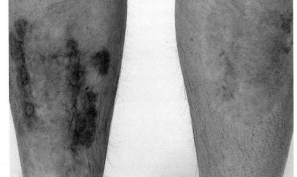

329 Healing necrobiosis lipoidica leaves an unsightly scar.

330

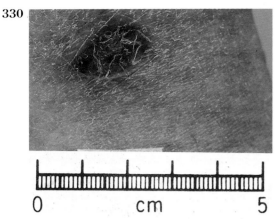

330 Diabetic dermopathy occurs mainly on the shins. The lesion is initially erythematous but later becomes atrophic and hyperpigmented. Intimal thickening of small blood vessels is the probable aetiology.

3

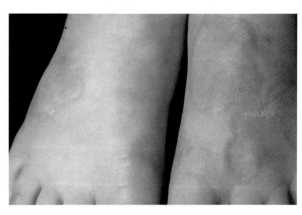

331 Granuloma annulare presents as a papular rash in annular or crescentic configurations mainly over the extensor surfaces of fingers but also feet, ankles, hands and wrists. Pathology is similar to necrobiosis lipoidica and may be associated with covert or overt diabetes.

332

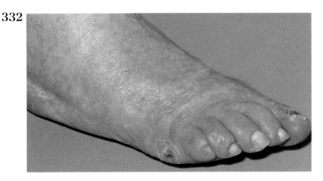

332 Diabetic foot with ischaemic ulcer on lateral border of distal end of the fifth metatarsal.

3

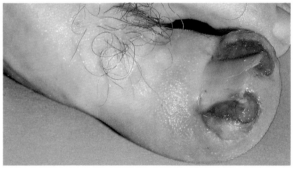

333 Ingrowing toenails in diabetic patients can often lead to severe infections. Proper chiropody can prevent this.

334

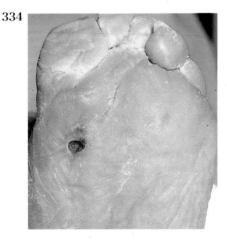

334 Neuropathic ulcer on the ball of the foot due to friction, with subsequent infection associated with an untreated corn. Note the severe tinea pedis (Athlete's foot) infection between the toes.

3

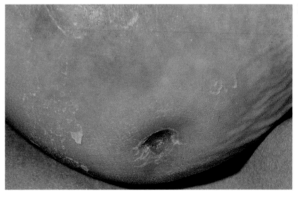

335 Heel ulcer. This is another common site for an ischaemic ulcer in a diabetic patient.

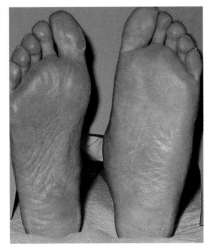

336 Charcot left foot. Neuropathy resulted in the development of a disorganised foot which was painless but markedly swollen and erythematous.

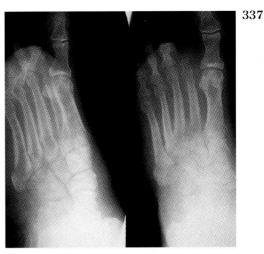

337 Osteomyelitis of metatarsals in a diabetic foot. The radiograph on the left shows the foot on first presentation with the metatarsals intact. On the right the infection has eroded away the proximal ends of the middle metatarsals and involved the adjoining tarsal bones.

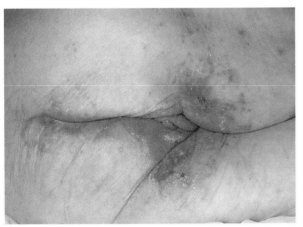

338 Candidiasis of buttock cleft and perineum with satellite lesions in an obese, diabetic patient.

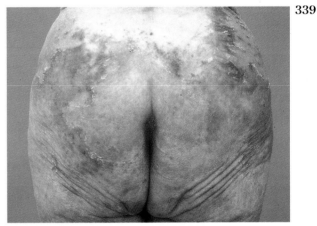

339 Glucagonoma rash in an obese, diabetic woman. It is described as a necrolytic, migratory erythema, often beginning in the buttock cleft or perineum as an erythematous rash which spreads outwards, progressing to bullae which break down with crust formation.

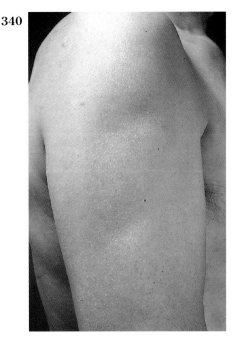

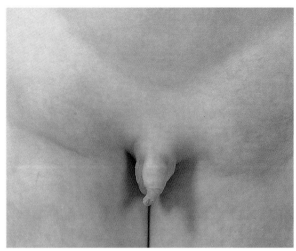

341 Lipodystrophy is hypertrophy of subcutaneous fat at sites of insulin injection. The absorption of insulin from such sites can be unpredictable.

340 Diabetic lipoatrophy involves an immune reaction to some contaminant of commercial insulin. It improves if highly purified insulins are used.

342

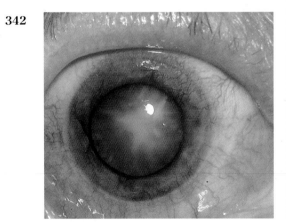

343

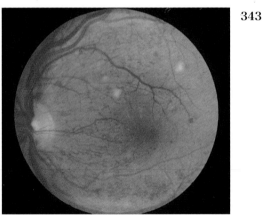

344

342 Rubeosis of the iris and cataract. New blood vessels grow onto the surface of the iris eventually causing glaucoma. Cataracts are common in diabetics and this is an advanced 'senile' type.

343 Proliferative diabetic retinopathy. There is extensive new vessel formation, blot haemorrhages and soft exudates.

344 Proliferative diabetic retinopathy. New vessels grow into the vitreous and may haemorrhage as can be seen next to the optic disc.

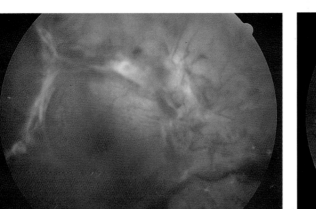

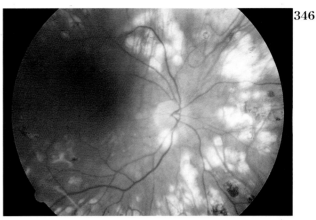

345 Vitreous haemorrhage, end-stage scarring and detachment are the result of end-stage, untreated, diabetic retinopathy. Vitrectomy surgery may restore some visual function.

346 Laser burns were successfully used to treat new vessel formation in this diabetic fundus.

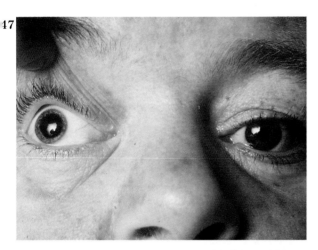

347 Oculomotor palsy. This produces ptosis of the right eye. With the eyelid elevated the dilated pupil is clearly seen and the eye is permanently abducted. Palsy of the third, fourth and sixth cranial nerves may occur with only mild diabetes. Improvement is often seen within a month.

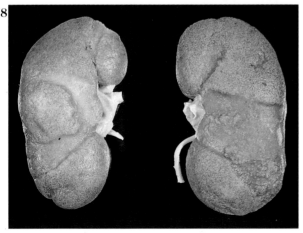

348 Diabetic kidneys. Note the cortical scarring due to glomerulosclerosis and recurrent pyelonephritis.

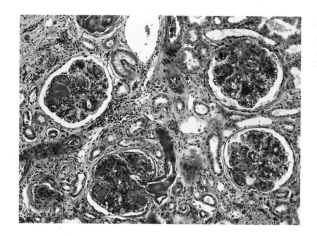

349 Diabetic nephropathy. Kimmelsteil-Wilson lesions are seen as rounded, acellular, hyaline nodules in the glomerular tufts. There is extensive deposition of hyaline material in Bowman's capsule and in the arterioles.

350

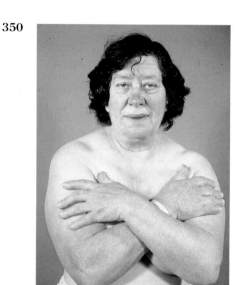

351

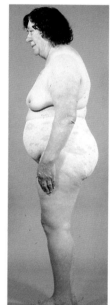

350 Acromegalic diabetic. This obese woman was noted as having diabetes but closer examination of her facial features suggested acromegaly. Acromegaly does not predispose to obesity but the diagnosis should not be forgotten in an obese diabetic with coarse features, excessive perspiration and lethargy.

351 Acromegalic facies of patient in **350** with thickened skin, coarse features and excessive sweatiness. Note the large hands.

9 Endocrinology, Hirsutism, Polycystic Ovarian Syndrome and Gynaecomastia

Hirsutism

When a female has an amount of hair on her face, body or limbs which is inappropriate for the race to which she belongs or the culture in which she lives, she is said to suffer from hirsutism. Hirsutism is prevalent in obese women possibly as a consequence of polycystic ovarian syndrome. Recent studies suggest that hirsutism, even in women with regular menstrual cycles, may in fact represent a part of the spectrum of polycystic ovarian syndrome. The rarer causes of hirsutism are shown in **Table 32**. Virilisation is a male pattern of hair distribution with temporal balding, breast atrophy, deepening of the voice and clitoromegaly. This may occur in women with severe hirsutism and is an indication of highly elevated androgen production due to more serious pathology.

Table 32. Causes of Hirsutism

Most common:	Polycystic ovarian syndrome	
Rarer causes:	Ovary	Hyperthecosis
		Hilus cell hyperplasia
		Virilising tumours (e.g. arrhenoblastoma)
	Adrenal	Congenital adrenal hyperplasia
		Adrenal adenoma/carcinoma (e.g. Cushing's)
	Drugs	Anabolic steroid
		Danazol
		Phenytoin
		Minoxidil
		Diazoxide

Management in the Obese

Weight loss can be efficacious in the hirsute obese and should be recommended. Where hirsutism is well localised, for example on the face, local treatment is useful such as shaving using an electric razor, bleaching, depilatory creams and electrolysis. There are three forms of endocrine therapy, namely glucocorticoids, oral oestrogen or progesterone preparations, and antiandrogenic drugs.

Glucocorticoids are used to suppress adrenal androgen output and as such are effective in congenital adrenal hyperplasia but are of little use in the management of the hirsute, obese woman. Oral oestrogen-progesterone preparations suppress ovarian androgen output but are of only minor benefit. This is possibly not surprising for most contain either norethisterone or norgesterel which themselves have endogenous, androgenic properties.

The most effective form of therapy is the anti-androgen, cyproterone acetate, available in the UK but not the USA. This compound not only blocks androgen receptors but also suppresses androgen productions. Side-effects vary but weight gain and lethargy are common. It is usually given with an oestrogen preparation to provide effective contraception for it would feminise a male fetus and teratogenicity cannot be excluded. Spironolactone has been used as an anti-androgen but it is considerably less efficient than cyproterone at removing unwanted hairs. With the recent reports of cancer in animals spironolactone has been withdrawn as a therapy for hirsutism in the UK.

Polycystic Ovarian Syndrome

The polycystic ovarian syndrome includes oligomenorrhoea, amenorrhoea and anovulatory menses, hirsutism and obesity associated with the finding of bilateral sclerocystic ovaries. Typically, serum levels of the androgens, testosterone and androstenedione, are elevated with a raised serum LH level in comparison to a normal or low FSH giving rise to an elevated LH to FSH ratio (often greater than 2.5).

The major source of the excess androgen appears to be the ovary, although there is evidence in some for excess adrenal androgen secretion. The exact pathogenesis of polycystic ovarian syndrome is not yet elucidated clearly but the low FSH is thought to play a major role in the failure of follicular maturation and persistent anovulation, since both can be rectified by exogenous FSH or antioestrogens which raise endogenous FSH levels.

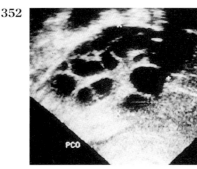
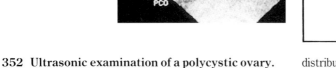

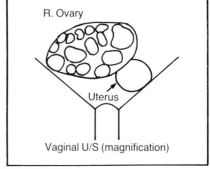

352 Ultrasonic examination of a polycystic ovary. The ovary is enlarged and contains many follicles, distributed mainly peripherally around an increased core of stroma.

353 Hirsutism in polycystic ovarian syndrome involving the upper lip, sides of face, chin and neck.

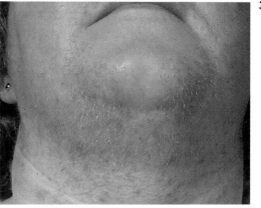

354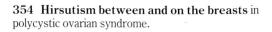

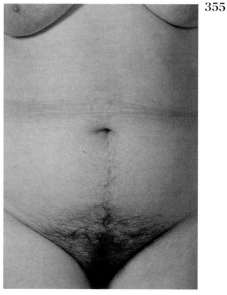

354 Hirsutism between and on the breasts in polycystic ovarian syndrome.

355 Hirsutism of linea alba as far as the umbilicus. This patient's excess weight, i.e. mild obesity, is typical of many patients with polycystic ovarian syndrome.

356 Hirsute abdomen of a male distribution is a severe feature in some patients with polycystic ovarian syndrome. These women can show a degree of virilism.

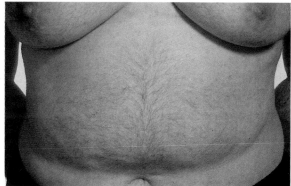

357 In Cushing's syndrome the degree of hirsutism can be variable. In this patient it extended over the upper lip, side of the face and chin. Note that the scalp hair has receded from the frontal and temporal areas.

358 Enlarged clitoris would be indicative of a more serious pathology in a hirsute woman.

357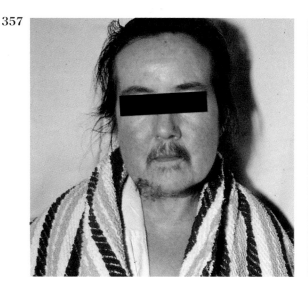

358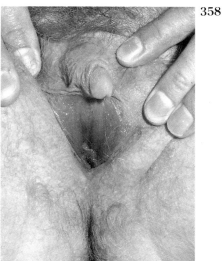

Gynaecomastia

Gynaecomastia is palpable, glandular breast tissue in men but often it is not easy to differentiate this clinically from fatty enlargement. This is important as in obesity men often exhibit enlarged breasts owing to increased fatty tissue. Nevertheless, in assessing whether glandular breast tissue is increased in an obese man with gynaecomastia one has to remember that palpable glandular tissue has been reported in up to 36% of normal males between the ages of seventeen and eighty years. Breast enlargement is considered a physiological rather than a pathological event in the newborn, at puberty, and in old age. Furthermore, breast enlargement can often occur with nutritional supplementation in a malnourished individual or on recovery from a severe illness when weight is regained.

Visible enlargement of neonatal breast in a fat baby is usually a manifestation of the normal physiological breast enlargement seen in newborns resulting probably from the action of maternal and/or placental oestrogens. This condition often settles in a month or so. Transient enlargement of the breasts is a normal occurrence in up to 40% of pubertal boys, the breasts often being asymmetrical and tender. By the age of twenty years most have setttled, although severe degrees, known as pubertal macromastia, can persist into adulthood. The cause is thought to be altered ratios of testosterone to oestrogen synthesis in the leydig and sertoli cell before testosterone-synthesising machinery has completed full development, or increased peripheral conversion of adrenal androgen to oestrogen before testosterone formation by the testes reaches a zenith.

The third occasion when glandular tissue gynaecomastia may be physiological in an obese male is during the sixth or later decades of life. Forty per cent of elderly males have been reported to have true glandular gynaecomastia, again due possibly to alterations with age in the testosterone to oestrogen ratio within breast cells.

In obese men who develop true glandular gynaecomastia between the ages of 20 and 60 years, or whose pubertal gynaecomastia fails to regress, one should investigate for underlying endocrine cause. Nevertheless, published series indicate that in 75% of such individuals no underlying endocrinopathy is found. **Table 33** shows the common pathological causes. One should note the many drugs which have been implicated. If the gynaecomastia is solely or mainly due to fat, weight loss in the obese man definitely is helpful, but where excess glandular tissue is involved plastic surgery is often necessary.

Gynaecomastia is said to be a risk factor for malignancy of the breast in men but this risk appears to be very slight. In one series, where 228 patients with gynaecomastia were followed up for ten years, not one developed breast cancer.

Some women with obesity can experience massive breast development due to fat deposition. This has to be distinguished from true hypertrophy which can also be seen in lean women. Here the enlargement can be due to multiple fibroadenomatous tissue or to diffuse lipomatosis (ref. 39, 40, 41).

Table 33. Causes of True Glandular Gynaecomastia	
Physiological	Neonatal
	Pubertal
	Senescent
	Renutrition following malnourishment
Pathological	Idiopathic (75%)
	Testosterone deficiency
	e.g. Kallman
	Noonan
	Panhypopituitarism
	Klinefelter's
	Sertoli cell only syndrome
	Viral orchitis
	Oestrogen excess
	Thyroid disease
	Liver disease
	Adrenal disease
	Testicular tumours
	Bronchial tumours
	Drugs
	Oestrogen, spironolactone, digoxin, ketaconazole, cimetidine, methyldopa, marijuana, heroin

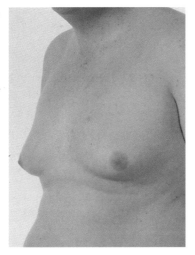

359 Marked gynaecomastia in a mildly obese, middle-aged patient not due to any definable endocrinopathy.

360 Adolescent gynaecomastia is due to pubertal physiological development and often regresses.

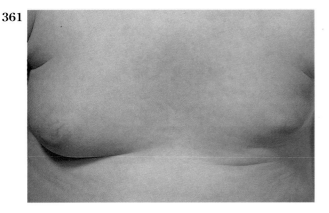

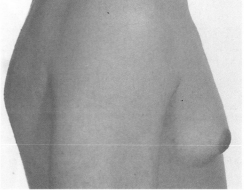

361 Premature thelarche in a two year old overweight girl. This is an extreme variation of normal possible due to slight secretion of oestrogen by the ovary.

362 Primary hypothyroidism. Gynaecomastia of glandular tissue in an adolescent which did not regress after puberty. Subsequent studies showed primary hypothyroidism. Gynaecomastia is more commonly noted in thyrotoxicosis than hypothyroidism.

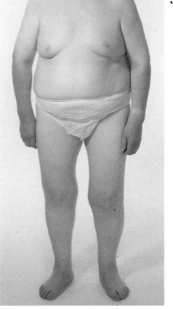

363 Frohlich-type, adult dwarf. This middle-aged man had suffered from partial hypopituitarism since he was a boy but regrettably this had not been recognised. He was of short stature with marked features of secondary hypothyroidism and hypogonadism. Note the gynaecomastia and obesity.

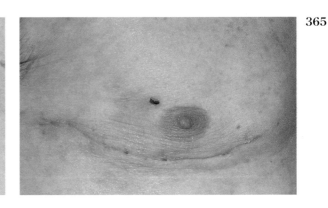

364 Operation. Often the only remedy for painful gynaecomastia is to remove the breast tissue.

365 Postoperative result in patient in **364** using an inframammary approach.

366

367

368

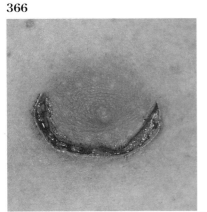

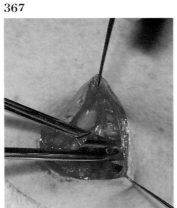

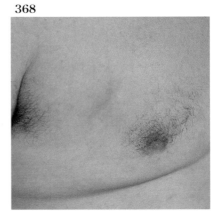

366 & 367 Periareolar incision (**366**) with subsequent dissection of breast tissue (**367**).

368 Postoperative result in a patient who had a periareolar incision for removal of gynaecomastic tissue induced by spironolactone.

Neuroendocrine Function in Obesity

369 Growth hormone (GH) response to insulin hypoglycaemia. Obese subjects usually show poor GH response to insulin hypoglycaemia which contrasts with that observed in muscular (non obese) individuals of similar weight. Therefore weight alone is not the cause of the reduced GH response (ref. 42).

TrS = Triceps skinfolds

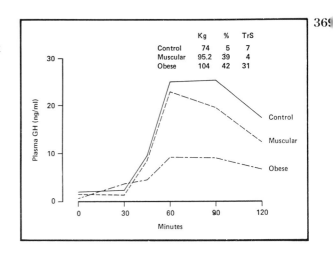

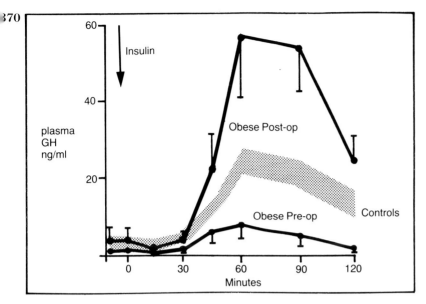

370 The abnormal growth hormone response to insulin hypoglycaemia seen in the obese state was corrected with substantial weight loss following surgery, suggesting that this abnormality is a consequence rather than a cause of obesity (ref. 43).

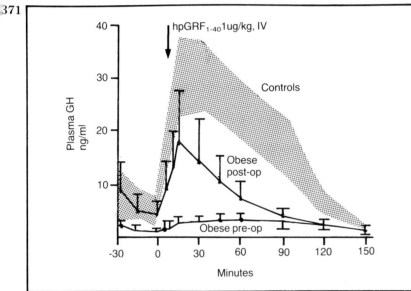

371 Impaired GH response to growth hormone releasing factor (GRF). A similar impaired response to GRF is also observed with a close correlation to the degree of obesity. In this study by Williams and colleagues the GH response to GRF improved with weight loss after surgery. It has been conjectured that with excess energy intake leading to obesity, somatostatin is released accounting for the impaired GH response to insulin hypoglycaemia and to GRF (ref. 43).

372 Thyrotrophin (TSH) response to thyrotrophin releasing hormone (TRH) is only reduced when weight gain becomes massive (ref. 44).

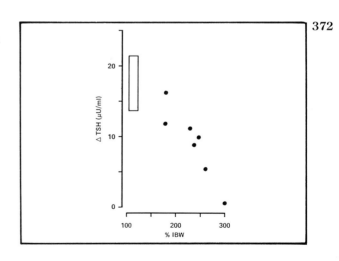

373

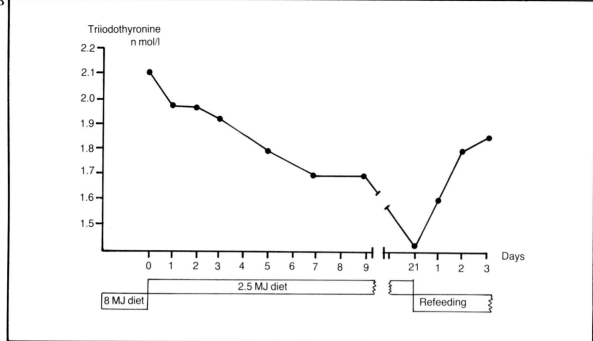

373 Serum triiodothyronine (T$_3$) levels are dependent on energy input, especially carbohydrate intake. Triiodothyronine decreases on a low energy diet, returns to pre-diet levels on refeeding and increases further on overfeeding. This dependency on energy intake possibly accounts for the various levels of serum triiodothyronine described in obesity. Serum thyroxine is unaltered by energy intake whereas reverse T$_3$ shows reciprocal changes, rising on dieting and decreasing on overfeeding (ref. 45).

374

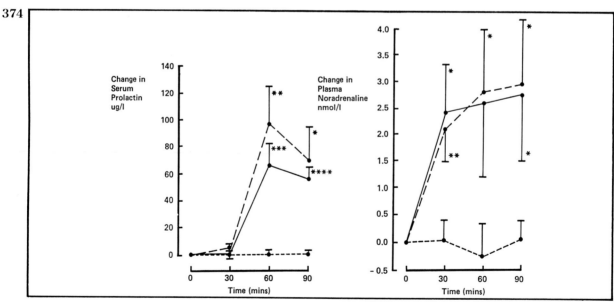

374 Prolactin response is variable. There are two distinct patterns in obesity. Some show no prolactin response to insulin hypoglycaemia (the non-responders) whereas others have a normal rise (the responders). Noradrenaline usually rises in response to hypoglycaemia. This is not observed in the prolactin non-responders, suggesting a link between the endocrine hypothalamic alteration in these obese subjects and the sympathetic nervous system, important in the control of energy expenditure. The prolactin response to TRH is usually normal in the hypoglycaemia non-responders.

Lean women ●————●
post-obese responders ●- - - - -●
post-obese non-responders ●············●

*p < 0.05, **p < 0.02, ***p < 0.01, ****p < 0.001 (ref. 46).

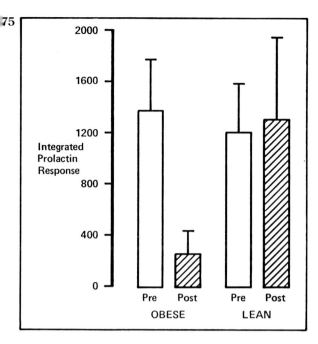

375 Conversion of prolactin responders to non-responders. The composition of the diet can alter the prolactin response to hypoglycaemia. An isocaloric, high carbohydrate diet for just one week impaired the prolactin response to hypoglycaemia in previously obese prolactin responders. Nevertheless, a similar isocaloric diet in lean women did not blunt the prolactin response. Hence, high carbohydrate intake alone, without any alteration in total caloric intake, can convert an obese prolactin responder to a non-responder with no appreciable weight change. This suggests that the prolactin abnormality in obesity is secondary to the nutritional intake, although the lack of change in the lean subjects also suggests that the obese subjects are in some way more 'susceptible' to nutritional change. Whether this susceptibility is inherited is debatable (ref. 47).

Table 34. Mean total and free levels of testosterone and oestradiol in obese males.

Body weight	Testosterone ng/ml	Free testosterone pg/ml	Oestradiol pg/ml	Free oestradiol fg/ml
Lean	6.22	125	25.4	505
140-170%	5.28	121	28.7	552
170-200%	4.25	117	37.9	779
> 200%	2.54	93	44.7	992

Table 34. Serum total testosterone decreases with obesity especially in those more than 200% of their ideal weight. Despite this there are usually no clinical signs of hypogonadism as the serum binding protein for testosterone, SHBG, also decreases with obesity maintaining the free and active testosterone level.

Nevertheless, in the most obese, free testosterone does decrease. In those over 200% of their ideal weight some have described hypogonadotrophic hypogonadism, suggesting a reduced LHRH drive. Both total and free serum oestradiol increases with obesity in males (ref. 48).

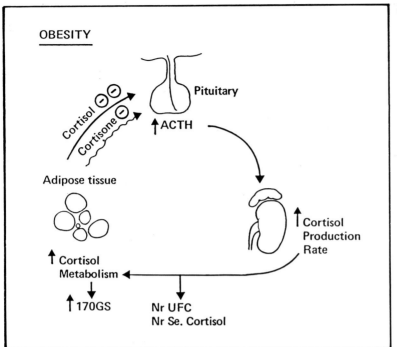

OBESITY

Cortisol ⊖ ⊖
Cortisone ⊖

Pituitary

↑ACTH

Adipose tissue

↑Cortisol Production Rate

↑Cortisol Metabolism ◄

↑17OGS   Nr UFC
           Nr Se. Cortisol

376 Glucocorticoid response. Obese subjects usually have normal circulating, serum-cortisol levels with a normal serum-cortisol circadian rhythm and normal urinary-free cortisol (UFC). Nevertheless, there is an accelerated degradation of cortisol, resulting in increased levels of cortisol degradation products, measured in urine as 17 hydroxycorticosteroids (17OGS). This increased degradation is compensated by an increased cortisol production rate, hence, plasma-cortisol levels remain unaltered. It has been suggested that the initial event is the enhanced metabolism of cortisol possibly in adipose tissue.

Obese subjects have a shift in the catabolism of cortisol to cortisone and one theory suggests that, as cortisone suppresses pituitary secretion of ACTH to a lesser degree than cortisol, the elevated cortisol production rate rises. This theory is still unproven and subject to discussion. Weight gain or loss is not required to alter the cortisol secretion rate for this can be achieved by alterations of caloric intake alone. Overfeeding lean volunteers elevates cortisol production rates. Fasting obese subjects for only 9 days will reverse the raised cortisol production rate.

Conclusion

Many of the neuroendocrine changes found in obesity are the consequences of the overfeeding which produces the obese state rather than of the obesity itself. It is conceivable that some obese individuals are, nevertheless, more susceptible to overfeeding than others. Whether this is an innate feature, or acquired owing to the timespan or degree of obesity, is not yet known.

10 Skin Lesions

Obesity is associated with striae, sweat rashes, yeast and fungal infections, boils and cellulitis. It is important to be able to distinguish such common complaints from more serious skin diseases, which at first sight may be overlooked as unimportant. Skin lesions linked with specific, obesity-associated diseases such as diabetes mellitus, lymphoedema, Cushing's myxoedema and acanthosis nigricans are illustrated elsewhere.

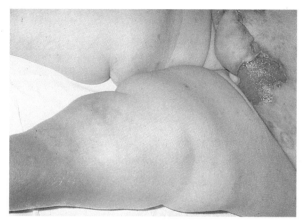

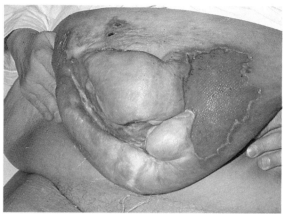

377 Cellulitis of left lower leg due to streptococcal infection.

378 Cellulitic abdominal apron. This apron became infected and eventually ulcerated, requiring operative apronectomy.

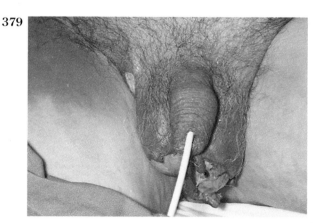

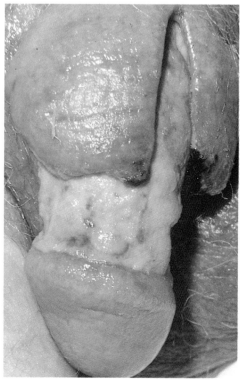

379 Fourniere's gangrene. Streptococci, in association with other organisms, set up a fulminating inflammation within the scrotal subcutaneous tissues, resulting in obliterative arteritis of the arterioles supplying the overlying skin. The scrotal coverings have sloughed.

380 Fourniere's gangrene involving the penile skin.

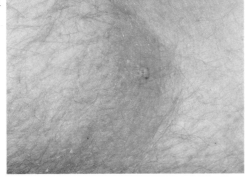

381

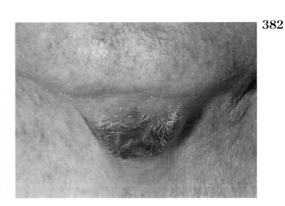

382

381 Furuncle. This is a staphylococcal infection of a hair follicle. This boil is beginning to point. Commonly found in neck, axilla, buttocks, groin and other hairy areas.

382 Carbuncle. Infective gangrene of subcutaneous tissues due to staphylococcal infection. Initially resembles a boil but spreads to deeper tissues and when rupture occurs there may be several skin openings. Found more often in males over 40 years of age in association with diabetes mellitus.

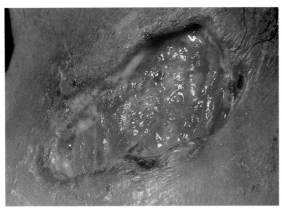

383 Carbuncle. Untreated result. The overlying skin of this infected area has sloughed leaving a large ulcer on this man's neck.

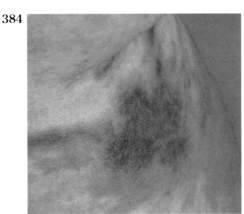

384

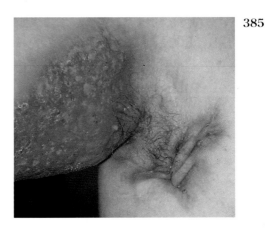

385

384 Cellulitis of axilla. This often arises in sweat-affected axillae.

385 Hidradenitis suppuratura. Boils in the axilla and groins can be the beginning of hidradenitis suppuratura, an intractable condition affecting the apocrine sweat glands. Firm, supporting nodules arise and coalesce, forming an indurating lesion punctuated by draining sinuses.

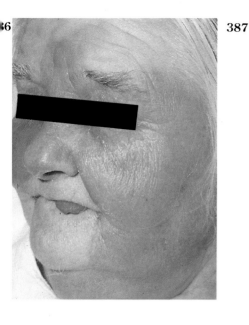

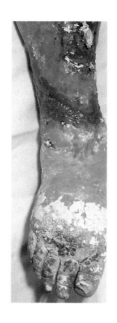

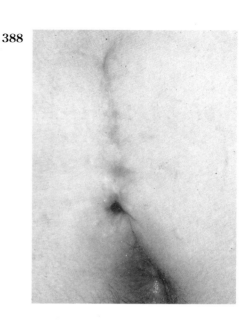

386 Facial erysipelas. Streptococcal facial cellulitis.

387 Lymphoedema, ulceration and cellulitis.

388 Pilonidal sinus at buttock cleft near the base of the coccyx. Purulent fluid, and occasionally loose hairs, can be expressed by pressure over the surrounding area. Similar lesions have been described at the interdigital clefts of fingers and at the umbilicus.

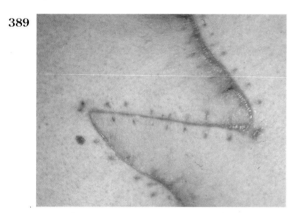

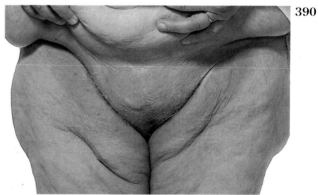

389 Pilonidal sinus Z repair.

390 Sweat rash underlying an apron of fat with involvement of the groins and perineum.

391 This **sweat rash**, underlying a large breast, was moist, irritable and clearly demarcated.

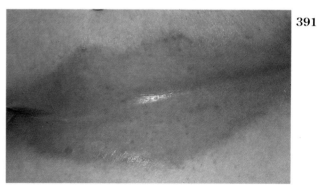

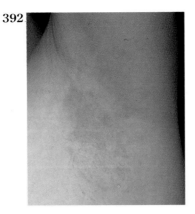

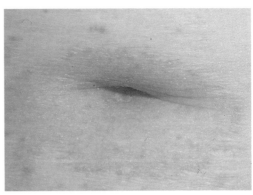

392 Moniliasis of axilla. Satellite vesico-pustules at the edge of the moist, infected area are highly suggestive of candidiasis (thrush). Candida favour damp, intertrigonous areas, especially in patients with diabetes mellitus.

393 Moniliasis of umbilicus. Note satellite lesions.

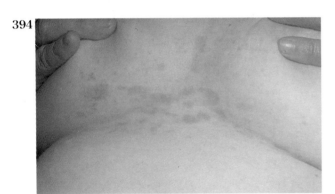

394 Moniliasis of breast. Sweat rashes under large breasts in fat women is common. Satellite lesions indicated that candida was the cause here.

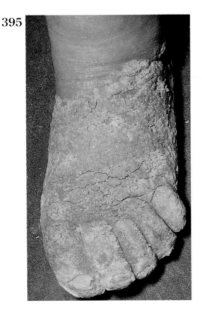

395 Chronic candidiasis of foot.

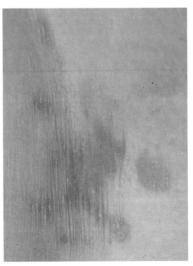

396 Psoriasis of axilla. Brief examination might confuse this with a candidal sweat rash of the axilla. In psoriasis the lesions consist of demarcated, pink areas of skin with silvery scaling as seen here.

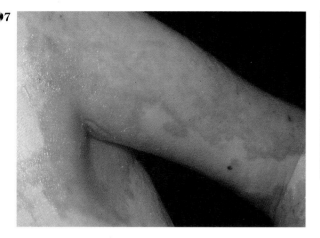

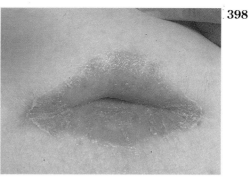

397 Psoriasis of axilla extending over arm and chest wall.

398 Psoriasis of umbilicus.

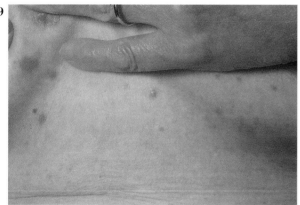

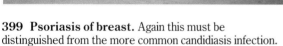

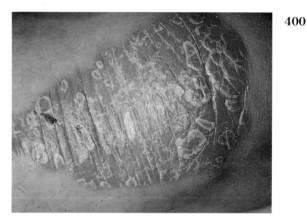

399 Psoriasis of breast. Again this must be distinguished from the more common candidiasis infection.

400 Psoriatic patch showing the sharp demarcation and silvery scaling.

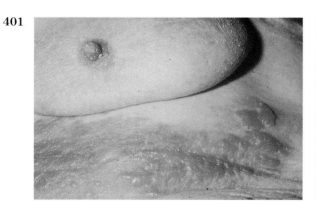

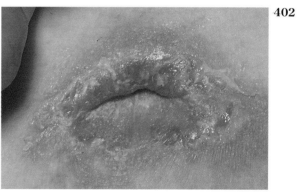

401 Shingles under breast.

402 Pemphigus of umbilicus. If this involves the upper epidermis, no blisters form and the lesion appears red and exudative. If it involves the deeper aspects of the epidermis, blisters do form.

403

403 Pemphigus affecting the lower thoracic wall underlying the breasts. Note the degree of exudation.

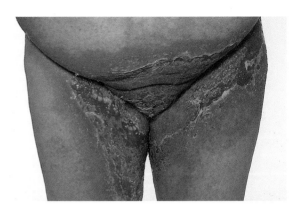

404 Pemphigus of groin and perineum. Pemphigus also involves the mucous membranes of vulva, mouth and pharynx and can present at these sites before skin lesions develop.

405

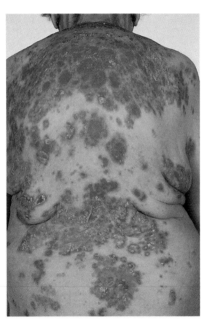

406

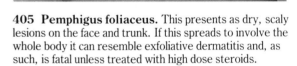

405 Pemphigus foliaceus. This presents as dry, scaly lesions on the face and trunk. If this spreads to involve the whole body it can resemble exfoliative dermatitis and, as such, is fatal unless treated with high dose steroids.

406 Dermatitis herpetiformis in region of the breasts. The eruption consists of urticarial papules and small groups of blisters. Itching is intense and the blisters are soon scratched open.

407

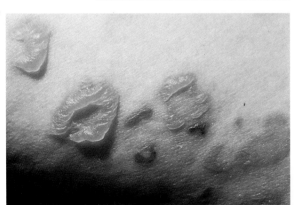

407 Dermatitis herpetiformis in close up, showing the papules and characteristic blisters. Most patients with this condition have an underlying gluten enteropathy (coeliac disease).

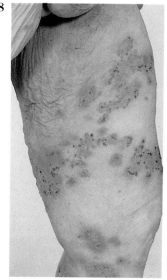
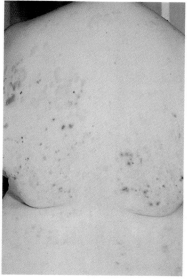
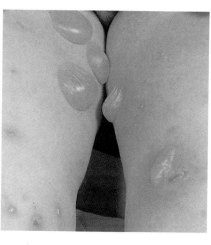

408 Dermatitis herpetiformis of groin, thigh and knee region. Pigmentation is often present where lesions have persisted for some time.

409 Dermatitis herpetiformis of back. This condition involves not only the upper back, but also the shoulders, sacrum, elbows, knees, buttocks and pressure areas.

410 Pemphigoid. Unlike pemphigus, the site of blister formation is at the basement membrane between the epidermis and the dermis. Hence, the blister's roof is thicker and less likely to rupture than in pemphigus. In contrast with pemphigus, the skin is usually first affected by a premonitory itching eruption which can resemble urticaria or eczema. Mucous membranes are affected little, if at all. Pemphigoid, if untreated, can run a chronic course over a matter of years and does not carry a high mortality rate like pemphigus. Treatment is with steroids.

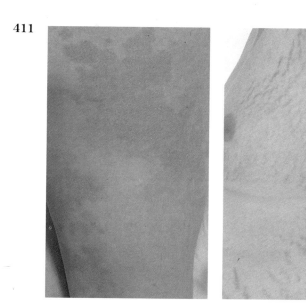

411 Urticaria of buttock and thigh due to salicylate.

412 Striae are often found in the obese, especially if they have rapidly gained weight. Stretch marks are also seen during the rapid growth phase of adolescence and during pregnancy. They are due to disruption of the dermal support tissue. Initially they are reddish-purple but later fade to an opalescent, white colour.

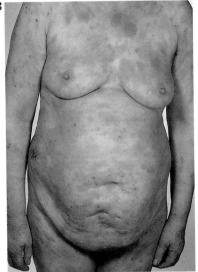

413 Mycosis fungoides. A reticulosis involving the skin. Infiltration of the skin and tumour formation are the final stages of this lymphoma, preceded by a variety of non-specific eczematous or psoriasiform eruptions associated with pruritus and lack of response to treatment.

414 Addision's disease. This obese patient suddenly began to lose weight, something the patient had found difficult to achieve in the past. A pigmentary ring was found encircling her abdomen in the region of her pant elastic. No buccal pigmentation was observed. She responded to steroid replacement, ironically regaining her obesity.

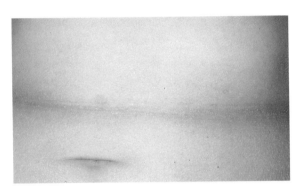

41

415

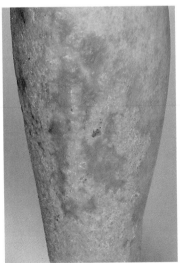

415 Hypertrophic lichen planus. Usually begins as an itching eruption on the wrists, spreading to the trunk and the legs. The lesions normally consist of purplish, flat-topped, shiny papules, polygonal in outline and often umbilicated. On the shins the lesions become warty, larger and form plaques.

416 Oral lichen planus. Mouth lesions can aid diagnosis. These may appear before the skin eruption or during its course. Delicate, white striae on the buccal mucosa are the most common presentation, although annular or dot lesions resembling candidiasis may appear.

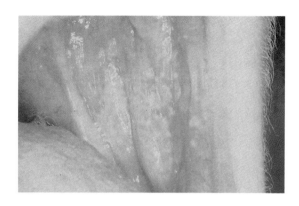

416

417

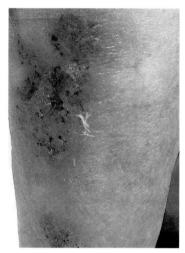

417 Pyoderma gangrenosum of skin. This condition is often associated with ulcerative colitis or Crohn's disease. The ulcers on the skin are multiple and cover large areas of the leg. The ulcers have ragged, blue-red, overhanging edges with necrotic bases. They often start as pustules or tender, red nodules following very minor trauma.

418 Pretibial myxoedema can occur in obese, thyrotoxic patients and at first sight suggest cellulitis. There are a number of varieties including a warty form, an oedematous form and a nodular type. This oedematous type gives rise to coarse, violaceous skin, thickened hair and non-pitting oedema.

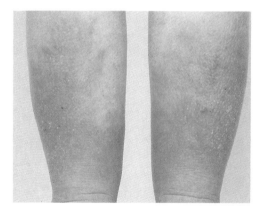

418

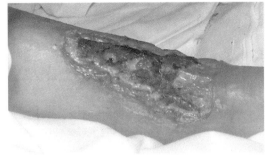

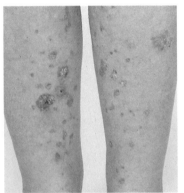

419 Arthritis ulcer. In this case due to a vasculitis associated with rheumatoid arthritis.

420 Vasculitis eruption — close up view.

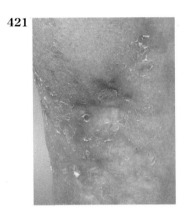

421 Bazin's disease. Also known as erythema induratum. The most common cause is active tuberculosis. The lesions can initially resemble severe chilblains. The lesion consists of deeply infiltrated plaques and nodules, cyanotic in colour, cold to touch and symmetrically situated on cold, blue areas of the calves. Some lesions ulcerate forming deep, 'punched out' ulcers. This condition usually develops in cold weather, improving and healing with scar formation in the summer. Antituberculous treatment is effective.

422 Solar keratosis of Bowenoid type. Sunlight can induce solar keratosis, characterised by small, red plaques covered with hard, irregular, abrasive scale. Bowen's disease, an intra-epidermal carcinoma of the skin, appears as eroded, beef-red plaques which are variably scaly and, as such, can resemble chronic eczema or psoriasis.

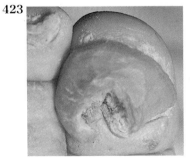

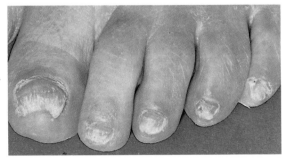

423 Onychogryophosis is due to hypertrophy of the nails.

424 Fungal infection of the nails.

11 Respiratory, Joint, Psychological and Obstetric Problems

Respiration

Obesity does affect the function of the lungs in a number of ways. The majority of obese patients have normal respiratory function tests and normal arterial carbon dioxide levels, but have abnormalities of ventilatory mechanics and gas exchange. A small number of very obese individuals present with Pickwickian syndrome in which there is hypoventilation, hypercapnia (raised arterial carbon dioxide levels) and hypersomnolence.

To understand the respiratory abnormalities of obesity it is important to know the normal, physiological respiratory responses in healthy, lean individuals. Normal, thin individuals' ventilation decreases during all stages of sleep. In non-rapid eye movement sleep (non-REM) ventilation decreases to 90-95% of the level observed during wakefulness. In the rapid eye movement (REM) phase of sleep, when one dreams, ventilation has been reported at about 84% of the level during wakefulness. Ventilation is usually increased by a low arterial oxygen level (hypoxia) or a raised arterial carbon dioxide concentration (hypercapnia). In normal individuals hypoxic ventilatory response is decreased during sleep, being lowest during the REM phase. This is more marked in the male than female. Hypercapnic ventilatory response also decreases during sleep, falling significantly in the non-REM phase with a further decrease in REM sleep to about one-third of the level during wakefulness. Hypoxia appears to be a poor stimulus to arousal as normal subjects remain asleep when arterial oxygen saturation has fallen as low as 70%. There is no difference in this respect between the REM and non-REM sleep phases. Hypercapnia is only slightly more potent than hypoxia in inducing arousal, most normal subjects being aroused before the arterial carbon dioxide level has risen by 15 mmHg above the level during wakefulness.

Obese Patient

Respiratory mechanics when awake

Too much fat in the chest wall and abdomen alters the mechanical properties of respiration. Hence, an increased respiratory muscle force is necessary to overcome the elastic recoil effect of the extra fat, especially when an obese person lies flat. A similar situation can be mimicked in thin individuals with weights attached to their chest. Most obese subjects respond by increasing the muscular activity of the diaphragm, which shows a response to hypercapnia nearly four times greater than that seen in normal weight individuals. Thus, most obese individuals appear to overcome the effect of the extra fat weight.

However, there are some who do not, namely those with the obesity hypoventilation syndrome (**Pickwickian syndrome**). When a normal, thin individual changes from the sitting to the lying position, vital capacity and expiratory reserve volume decrease. This is accentuated in obesity, especially in those with the obesity hypoventilation syndrome.

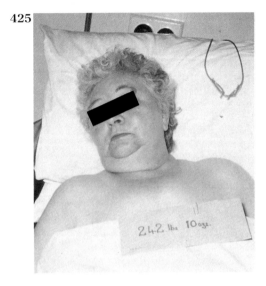

425

425 Pickwickian syndrome. Daytime hypersomnolence in an obese patient due to the obesity-hypoventilation syndrome. This is often known as the Pickwickian syndrome in honour of the somnolent, fat boy, Joe, in Charles Dickens' 'Pickwick Papers'. Note that the nasal prongs used to provide oxygen should be applied to the patient!

Gas exchange when awake

In severe obesity there is also a disturbance of ventilation-perfusion balance. Obese subjects have less ventilation to their well-perfused lower lobes in comparison to healthy, thin individuals. This abnormality is most marked in those obese subjects with the greatest decrease in expiratory reserve volume. Hence, the lower portions of the lungs in the obese are relatively underventilated and overperfused. This is manifested by varying degrees of hypoxia, but normal arterial carbon dioxide levels. The hypoxia is accentuated if the obese patient lies flat. There appears to be a sex difference in that this hypoxic effect is seen in males and not often in premenopausal females. Possibly the male, abdominal distribution of fat is the important factor.

Respiration during sleep

Sleep apnoea/hypoventilation syndrome is found in normal weight individuals, but is more prevalent in the obese. In this syndrome the subject has periods of apnoea (i.e. no breathing) lasting longer than 10 seconds on at least 15 occasions per hour of sleep. Alternatively, the subject exhibits episodes of hypopnoea resulting in at least 15 episodes of arousal per hour of sleep. These episodes must be associated with supporting symptoms for diagnosis of this syndrome to be confidently made. The symptoms are usually restless sleep, grunting respiration, snoring and daytime somnolence. Morning headaches, decreased libido, impotence and enuresis are also possible symptoms. The medical sequelae are more difficult to define but arrhythmias are common during apnoeas which are also associated with mild systemic hypertension. Coexisting, daytime hypoventilation with hypoxia also results in secondary polycythaemia, cor pulmonale and pulmonary hypertension.

It is only in recent years that the prevalence of this syndrome has been appreciated. The suggested prevalence in the population in general has been reported as 1%. Research on seemingly healthy, obese subjects indicates a much greater prevalence than hitherto thought, even in those with normal respiration whilst awake. If the obese individual already shows daytime hypoxia the normal physiological changes during REM sleep will result in further hypoxaemia. This has pathophysiological importance as the hypoxic complications mentioned previously relate to the absolute level of arterial oxygenation.

The apnoeic or hypoventilatory episodes during sleep can have an obstructive, central or mixed aetiology. In obstructive apnoea, the obstruction occurs in the pharynx and is associated with a loss of tone of the pharyngeal and glossal muscles. The relaxation of the genioglossus allows the base of the tongue to fall back against the posterior pharyngeal wall and occlude the pharynx. In central apnoea, the brain's respiratory centre is involved, although often a central abnormality is associated with obstructive apnoea which only becomes apparent when the obstructive component is relieved by tracheostomy.

In the **obesity-hypoventilation syndrome** there is a marked depression in both hypercapnic and hypoxic respiratory drives. There are also marked apnoeic episodes both during sleep and the waking state. The apnoea can be obstructive, central or of mixed pattern. Sleep in these patients is frequently interrupted by arousal following apnoeic episodes. This apnoea worsens with increasing obesity, eventually resulting in such a degree of sleep deprivation that daytime hypersomnolence supervenes. The noctural hypoventilation is thought to alter respiratory control adversely, resulting in daytime hypoxia and hypercapnia with eventual pulmonary arterial hypertension, cor pulmonale (right-sided cardiac failure) and secondary polycythaemia. Persistent hypoxia further blunts the hypoxic ventilatory drive, leading to a vicious circle of events.

Weight loss greatly improves the condition of such patients, although the apnoeic syndrome may persist. Some have suggested that it is the susceptibility to apnoeic episodes which produces the obese-hypoventilation syndrome in some obese patients and not in others, despite similar degrees of obesity.

Investigations in the Obese

History can be helpful.

Most patients with **central apnoea** are symptomless but if the apnoea is prolonged it can result in the patient awakening with a panic attack or morning headaches. Insomnia may occur and poor night-time sleeping produces daytime lethargy.

In **obstructive apnoea** the patients often snore loudly, have disturbed, restless sleep and experience daytime tiredness. Depression and personality changes can occur.

Investigations

Overnight admission to a sleep unit is the best way to diagnose the situation effectively. Those without such a facility could use daytime and overnight ear lobe oximetry.

426

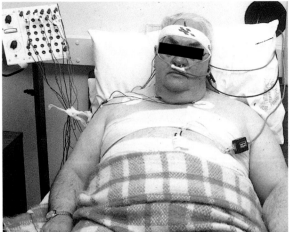

426 Sleep study. Complete study includes measurement of oxygen saturation, arterial carbon dioxide, airflow at nose and mouth, chest and abdominal movements, EEG, EMG, ECG and eye movement recordings.

427

DESATURATION IN SLEEP APNOEA IS GREATEST
DURING REM

427 Sleep study or oximeter readings during various phases of sleep show desaturation is maximal during REM phases.

428

428 On ward oximetry. Simple ear lobe measurements of arterial oxygenation using an oximeter can produce valuable information even in the most unsophisticated ward. In this case significant oxygen desaturation occurred.

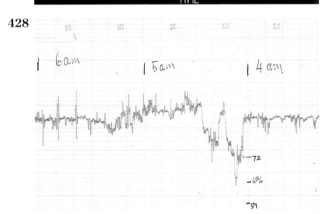

42

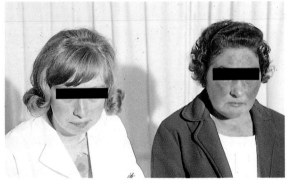

429 Secondary polycythaemia in the patient on the right as compared with a normal weight, non-polycythaemic woman on the left.

Management

Substantial weight loss is mandatory and is effective. In those with marked **obstructive apnoea**, any underlying cause should be treated. In some patients, relief of a nasal obstruction or removal of tonsils, adenoids or retropharyngeal masses may be helpful. One should exclude hypothyroidism since pharyngeal myxoid tissue may precipitate obstructive apnoea. Similarly, acromegaly ought to be excluded and the patient should avoid sedatives and alcohol. There are probably no longer any indications for tracheostomy in patients with obstructive apnoea, this therapy having been supplanted by continual positive airways pressure (CPAP). CPAP not only increases the pressure within the airways, overcoming the tendency of the airways to collapse, but also reflexly stimulates upper airway opening muscles and raises functional residual capacity. CPAP involves the delivery of pressurised air into the pharynx through a nasopharyngeal tube.

Drugs which alter pharyngeal tone or respiratory drive are used. Protryptyline reduces the amount of REM sleep and hence reduces the length of time during which obstruction may occur. Alcohol abstinence may be all that is required in some.

Table 35. Treatment of obesity hypoventilation syndrome

1. Substantial weight loss.
2. Exclude hypothyroidism, acromegaly — if present treat.
3. Avoid sedatives.
4. Alcohol abstinence.
5. ENT opinion — remove any obstruction.
6. Continual positive airways pressure.
7. Drugs — protryptilline
              medroxyprogesterone
8. Nocturnal oxygen.

Medroxy-progesterone, which acts as a respiratory stimulant, may be effective in some but by no means in all. Acetazolamide has also been reported as beneficial in some with central apnoea. An alternative treatment, which has found some favour, is nocturnal oxygen. Although oxygen may prolong some apnoeas it may decrease the number of apnoeic episodes and the amount of time spent apnoeic, hence improving sleep quality. Oxygen also raises the level of oxygenation during sleep with only a slight rise (< 1 mmHg) in the end-apnoeic carbon dioxide level. Arrhythmias are also reduced (ref. 49, 50).

Arthritis

Gout is a complication of obesity. The risk increases appreciably in males who are 130% or more above an average weight (100%). In middle-aged women the risk is 2.6-fold higher in those 180% or more in weight. Starvation-type diets can precipitate gout in those with hyperuricaemia.

Osteoarthritis is a more common condition than gout. Although the prevalence of arthritis in obesity is high, there are reports showing no correlation with the degree of obesity. Nevertheless, the study by Rimm and colleagues (ref. 28), of over 73,000 women in U.S.A. and Canada, did show that arthritis was related to obesity with a 1.55-fold higher risk in middle-aged women with severe obesity. Other studies have also shown a greater weight in those with osteoarthritis of weight-bearing joints together with an increase in obesity in those with osteoarthritis of the hands. The obese have also been reported to show radiological evidence of worse arthritic changes to the knee and hip joints. In elderly people, obesity and osteoarthritis may well be associated by chance, but arthritis, leading to reduced physical activity and hence weight gain, would appear to be one explanation for an interaction.

Weight reduction often reduces symptoms in various bone and joint diseases, especially if the bones and joints causing trouble are weight-bearing ones. Hence the importance of weight loss in the management of obese arthritis patients.

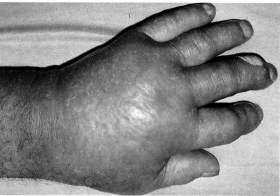

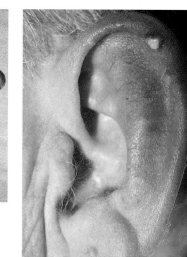

430 Gout. The hand in this patient is reddened, hot, swollen and exquisitely tender. Note the tophi on the second finger. Fifty % of those with gout in middle or late years are obese.

431 Ear lobe tophi. Urate deposit on the ear lobe. Twenty % of those with gout are said to have tophi.

432 Finger tophi.

433 Radiology of gouty hand. Note the 'punched out', radiolucent areas around the affected joints, especially noticeable on the distal phalangeal joint of the right index finger.

434 Gouty toe. The most commonly affected joint in 75% of cases is the metatarsophalangeal joint of the big toe.

435 Radiology of gouty toes. Note the radiolucent areas of the first metatarsal phalangeal joints of each big toe.

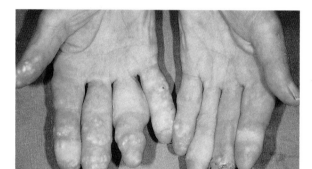

43

433

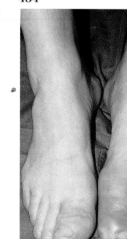

434

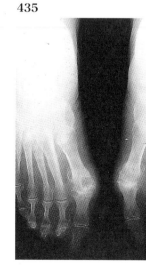

435

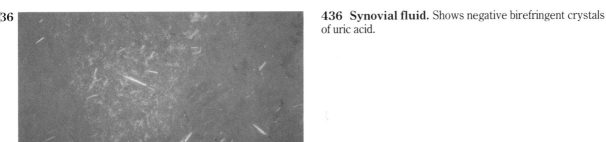

436 Synovial fluid. Shows negative birefringent crystals of uric acid.

437

438

439

437 Arthrogram showing a Baker's cyst which is a cystic swelling in the popliteal fossa (arrow), common in those with arthritic conditions of the knee.

438 Ruptured Baker's cyst. Rupture produced swelling and pain in the upper calf of the left leg. This can easily be mistaken for a deep, venous thrombosis.

439 Ruptured Baker's cyst. Contrast has leaked from the Baker's cyst producing the clinical picture shown in **438**.

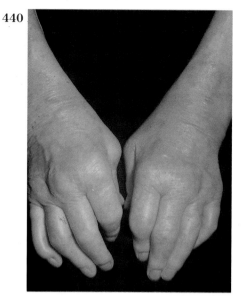

440 **Rheumatoid arthritis.** Typical features showing involvement of proximal interphalangeal and metacarpophalangeal joints. Weight loss in an obese patient with this condition can help to relieve the symptoms but it will not cure the condition.

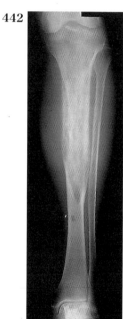

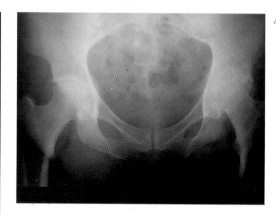

441 **Paget's disease** involving tibia. Obesity worsened the symptoms in this patient.

442 **Radiological changes in Paget's disease** of upper tibia. Note the sharp demarcation between the osteolytic pagetic front and normal bone.

443 **Osteoarthritis of left hip.** Cartilage space is diminished with sclerosis of the surface bone and osteophytic formation at the joint margins.

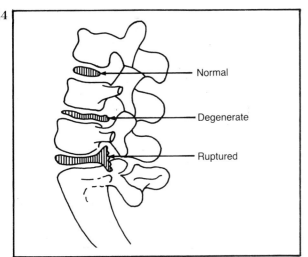

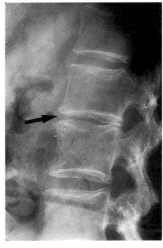

445

444 Lower back pain in the obese is often due to ruptured or degenerate intervertebral discs. This is often precipitated by injury but spontaneous age degeneration of the disc and obesity are important predisposing factors.

445 Radiology of lumbar spine showing vertebral disc collapse (arrow).

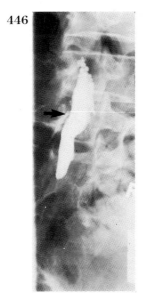

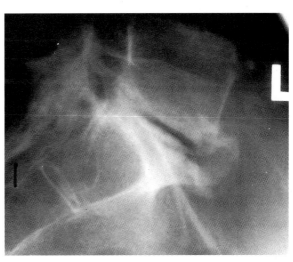

446 Myelogram showing central disc bulge (arrow) as an indentation of the column of intrathecal contrast.

447 Air in LS/S1 intervertebral disc which has degenerated and collapsed.

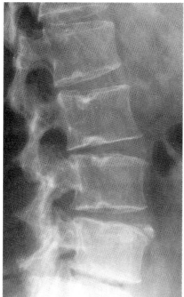

448 Schmorl's nodes shown on this radiograph are the consequence of the protrusion of a portion of the nucleosus pulposus of an intervertebral disc into adjoining bony vertebra. This is indicative of **osteoporosis** of the spine, which often results in vertebral collapse. Weight loss is essential in those obese subjects who develop this condition. Usually osteoporosis occurs in postmenopausal women, in whom oestrogen replacement halts the condition.

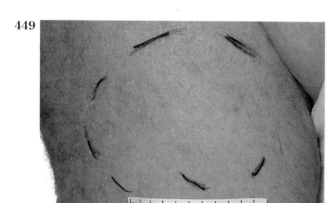

449 Meralgia paraesthetica in the obese is due to compression of the lateral cutaneous nerve of the thigh where it passes through or beneath the inguinal ligament. Pain and numbness are often precipitated by walking or standing, suggesting arterial or joint disease. The site of the pain is associated with relative anaesthesia of the skin of the outer aspect of the thigh shown here. Weight loss helps and can remit spontaneously. If the condition becomes troublesome, local anaesthetic infiltration, operative decompression or nerve division may be indicated.

Psychological Factors

It is widely recognised that obesity is associated with many psychological problems. Such problems may cause obesity, may be the result of obesity or may be the consequence of dieting. Food can be used as a substitute for affection or to relieve anxiety, boredom, frustration or even guilt. Psychological disturbances can range from mild feelings of inferiority to severe depression, especially in grossly obese women (25-30% incidence). In some there can be a severe distortion of body image and subjects often see themselves as being more obese than they are. This is especially seen on dieting. Some have reported that the psychological effects of obesity are most clearly seen when weight is reduced, with depression being the most commonly observed abnormality. Depression on dieting may be more a reflection of the way in which the weight loss is achieved rather than the weight loss itself since there is such variability in its incidence. Some actually observe a reduction in depressive scores. Many obese individuals are not obese as a result of psychological problems, rather these are often acquired as a consequence of developing obesity or dieting.

Operative Risks

Perioperative risks include difficulties with anaesthetic induction, the maintenance of anaesthesia and the postoperative recovery, especially with regard to respiration. The surgery itself may be technically difficult and associated with increased blood loss. Postoperatively, wound infection, deep vein thrombosis, pulmonary embolism, fluid imbalance and incisional hernias can be a major problem.

Pregnancy and Parturition

The most common obstetrical complication associated with obese women is an increased risk of hypertension. Diabetes mellitus, malpresentation, prolonged labour, post partum haemorrhage, post partum venous thrombosis and pulmonary embolism are all greater risks in the obese. Higher fetal weight has also been reported in obese women.

Renal

Forty per cent of obese subjects have been reported to have variable degrees of proteinuria, with only a small number having nephrotic syndrome. Glomerular abnormalities have been described in massive obesity. Glomerular size is augmented owing to capillary and arteriolar dilatation and can increase in cellularity, being mainly of mesangial origin with a small endothelial component. Modest hyperplasia of occasional juxta glomerular apparatuses has been reported as well as variable fat deposition in the cells of the tubules. Glomerulomegaly is possibly related to the increased blood volume of the obese, associated hypoxia and increased right ventricular pressure. In those with nephrotic syndrome, renal biopsy findings include focal and segmental glomerulosclerosis with fibrin like material deposition in the glomeruli. Whether this is directly due to obesity or to some other incidental but unidentifiable disease is debatable. Nevertheless, proteinuria diminishes in all patients with considerable weight reduction (ref. 51, 52).

450 Focal glomerulosclerosis in a renal biopsy from an obese patient with proteinuria. (PAS silver stain.)

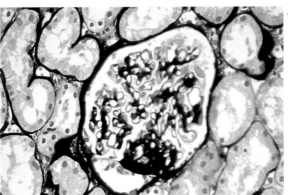

450

12 Treatment — Medical and Surgical

Table 36. Treatment Available	
Diet	standard diets
	very low energy diets
Physical activity	
Behavioural therapy	
Drugs	appetite suppressants
	thermogenic drugs
	fat absorption inhibition,
	e.g. tetrahydrolipstatin, DEAE-D
Surgery	jaw wiring
	gut bypass and gastroplasty
	gastric balloon
	apronectomy
	fat suction
Alternative medicine	

Table 37. Standard Diet
• Realistic energy intake
• Natural food
• Sound nutritional sense
• Education
• Weight loss goal

Diet

Aims

The major aims of a diet must be to re-educate the eating pattern of a patient and to encourage long-term compliance. To achieve this food must be palatable, easily available, inexpensive and the diet must be based on sound nutritional sense. Thus the diet should include:

- high fibre

- low fat

- sufficient carbohydrates, but in the form of starch rather than pure glucose or sucrose

- moderation in salt intake

- sufficient protein — a minimum of 80 g for a male and 60 g for a female

- adequate vitamins and minerals

- realistic energy intake

Energy in a Diet

In a reducing diet the particular energy requirements of the individual should always be assessed. For example:

1300 kcal (5.4 MJ) per day — most men will lose weight on this.

1000 kcal (4.2 MJ) per day — normally sufficient to produce weight loss in most men and women even after the intial decrease in basal metabolic rate.

800 kcal (3.31 MJ) per day — everyone will lose weight on this intake

Types of Standard Diet

List of acceptable and unacceptable foods

The patient has to have the willpower to avoid the non-acceptable foods. If the food desired is **not** on the list the patient may then consider it safe to consume even though the energy content could be high.

Menu style

This is more successful. The patient is given a detailed list of what they can eat and certain high energy containing foods are limited by weight. If the food is **not** on the menu it is **not** to be eaten. Educates and guarantees weight loss if kept to precisely.

Table 38. Menu style

Rules

- You must take breakfast and two main meals as detailed in the table.
- Milk allowance: 50 g dried skimmed milk or one pint fresh skimmed milk.
- Cooking: food must **not** be fried.
- One serving per day of low calorie soup is allowed.
- Free allowance of tea, coffee and low calorie drinks.
- Weigh food items shown.

Breakfast:	a. Half a grapefruit, or an orange or an apple, or 100 ml fresh, unsweetened orange juice. b. One slice (35 g) wholemeal bread.
Main Meals:	Two main meals are allowed, consisting of sections 1, 2 and 3 **and** one slice (35 g) of wholemeal bread at each meal.
Section 1.	Choose **one** of the following sources of protein. **Either** 60 g (cooked weight) lean meat, poultry or game **or** 100 g (cooked) white fish or shellfish e.g. cod, plaice, sole, haddock **or** 60 g (cooked) oily fish e.g. mackerel, salmon, herring **or** 100 g cottage cheese **or** 50 g hard, reduced fat cheese (max. 5 times weekly) **or** 2 eggs (max. 4 times weekly)
Section 2.	Choose unlimited quantities of any of the vegetables in Section A but, if you wish, also have 50 g of **one** of the vegetables in Section B. **Section A:** cabbage, cauliflower, lettuce, cucumber, runner or french beans, broccoli, brussel sprouts, marrow, celery, mushrooms, tomatoes, carrots, turnip, swede, onions, leeks, beansprouts. **Section B:** 50 g of peas, beans (haricot, butter, broad or red kidney), parsnips, beetroot, sweetcorn.
Section 3:	One piece of fruit, e.g. orange, apple, pear, peach **or** 120 g stewed apples **or** 100 g fresh pineapple, grapes, cherries **or** 150 g soft fruit i.e. strawberries, raspberries **or** unlimited stewed rhubarb.

Table 38 shows the Dundee '800' diet as used at Ninewells Hospital, Dundee, Scotland, under medical supervision (based originally, with modifications, on a diet devised by Professor W.P.T. James, reproduced with permission). A typical day's intake would provide 800 kcal (3.3 MJ), 64.6 g fat, 105.2 g carbohydrate, 20 g fibre and 58 mmol sodium.

Realistic Goals

- Reasonable weight loss for the first 6 weeks of an 800 (3.3 MJ) to 1000 (4.2 MJ) kcal diet for the average person is 1.5 lbs (0.65 kg) per week as both water and fat are lost.

- Subsequent weight loss will be slower and therefore, the target should be reduced to 1 lb (0.45 kg) per week.

- Always set a goal which is achievable.

- Remember **any** weight loss is an advantage even though ideal weight may never be achieved.

- Remember, once weight loss is achieved, a lifelong modification in eating habits is necessary to prevent regain.

Very Low Calorie Diets

- Minimum energy intake recommended:

  400 kcal (1.65 MJ per day — women under 173 cm (5 ft 8 ins) in height

  500 kcal (2.1 MJ) per day — for all men and for women over 173 cm (5 ft 8 ins) in height.

- Protein — good biological value
  > 50 g for males
  > 40 g for females

- Adequate minerals — prevent hypokalaemia

- Adequate vitamins

- Carbohydrates — essential that diet contains some to prevent excessive muscular protein breakdown to glucose.

Rules

- Maximum 6 weeks
- Under medical supervision

- Repeat no more than once in 3 months
- Cease if intercurrent illness develops

Contra-indications

Heavy smokers, alcoholics, unstable psychologically, cardiac abnormalities, including ischaemia and arrhythmias, infective and inflammatory diseases, abnormal liver, abnormal renal function.

Exercise

- Increases energy expenditure and promotes the development of lean tissue

- Relieves stress

- Produces feeling of well-being

- 30 minutes per day of brisk walking for one year with no specific diet will produce a 10 lb (4.5 kg) weight loss

- Build up gradually as too vigorous exercise initially in an obese, sedentary person could be unsafe

Table 39. To Lose 1 lb of Fat
Walk: 35 miles at 1 m.p.h.
Jog: 3.5 hours at 6 m.p.h.

Behavioural Therapy

This can be achieved through individual or group support. There are basically eight facets to this educational therapy. With **self monitoring** the patient keeps a diary of the type of food eaten, together with the place and time of consumption.

Stimulus control tries to prevent the patient eating in excess when food is presented. **Shopping** is recommended after eating, a list should be used and kept to and the patient is advised to avoid ready-to-eat food. Meal **plans** consist of eating at set times, not accepting food offered by others and substituting exercise for snacks. **Activities** include storing food out of sight, eating all food in the same place, leaving the table immediately after eating, possibly using smaller dishes and never saving leftovers. **Parties and holidays** should be planned in advance, taking low energy drinks, practising polite ways to decline food, possibly eating a low energy snack before a party and learning how to telephone the host/hostess to request a low energy meal.

Eating behaviour includes chewing thoroughly before swallowing, putting fork down between mouthfuls and not talking, reading or watching television while eating.

Table 40. Behavioural Therapy in Groups or Individually
• Self monitoring
• Stimulus control — shopping — planning — activity — parties and holidays
• Eating behaviour
• Reinforcement
• Cognitive restructuring
• Education
• Exercise
• Money factor

Reinforcement is rewarding oneself once goals are reached and soliciting help from family and friends.

Cognitive restructuring is to avoid unreasonable goals, to avoid imperatives such as 'never' and 'always', to think positively about achievements and progress and do not dwell on shortcomings.

Education and **exercise** are self explanatory. Finally, many groups use the reward of **money** to achieve success.

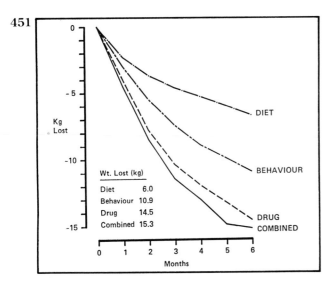

451 Behavioural therapy and weight loss. Stunkard and colleagues have shown that behavioural therapy with a diet results in improved weight loss compared with diet alone. Nevertheless, appetite suppressants such as fenfluramine result in a greater weight loss and behavioural therapy with fenfluramine provides no additional advantage (ref. 53).

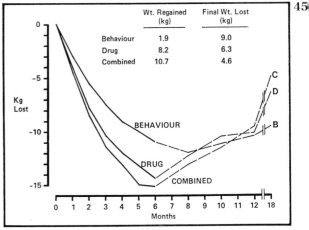

452 Behavioural therapy and weight gain. Behavioural therapy shows a marked advantage when weight regain is studied. Combined therapy with fenfluramine and behavioural modification apparently offers no advantage (ref. 53).

Table 41. Appetite Suppressants	
Phentermine Mazindol Diethylpropion	Affect catecholamine pathways
Fenfluramine Dex(tro)fenfluramine Fluoxetine	Affect serotonergic system

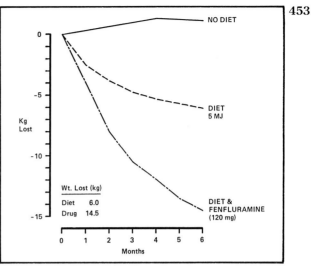

453 Fenfluramine and weight loss. In this work by Stunkard and colleagues, the appetite suppressant fenfluramine promoted weight loss. In other studies, the weight loss attributable to drug therapy is about 225 g per week. Once treatment is discontinued weight regain invariably occurs (Fig. **452**) (ref. 53).

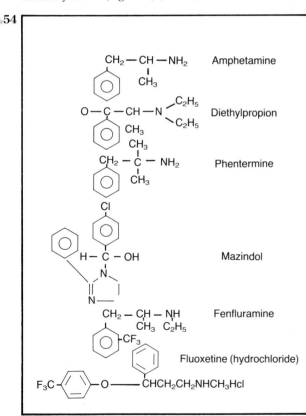

454 Chemical structure of anorectic drugs.
The chemically related compounds **phentermine** and **diethylpropion** reduced appetite through an action in the adrenergic neuroceptors in the brain. This anorectic effect is associated with central stimulation and euphoria and could be subject to abuse. However, addiction or dependency rarely occurs among patients who receive their drugs under medical supervision.
Fenfluramine promotes release of serotonin, enhancing satiety rather than directly reducing hunger. It has no stimulant action but can be associated with depression if the drug is stopped suddenly and, in some cases, has been associated with pulmonary hypertension.
Dex(tro)fenfluramine, the active isomer of fenfluramine, may be more efficacious.
Fluoxetine acts by blocking re-uptake of serotonin and is an effective anti-depressant associated with weight loss. This is quite unlike the tricyclic anti-depressants which produce weight gain.

157

Thermogenic Drugs

These drugs increase energy expenditure. **Thyroxine** and **triiodothyronine** have the disadvantage of causing severe loss of lean body mass. **L dopa**, used in Parkinson's disease, also promotes weight loss but has to be used in high dosages with consequent side effects. **Ephedrine** is converted to noradrenaline in the liver and, when given at a dosage of 60 mg per day for three months in women on a specific diet, has been reported to produce a 5.5 kg weight loss. Upward alterations of blood pressure and plasma glucose are a problem with acute dosages, but less of a problem when given chronically (ref. 54). **Methyl xanthine** derivatives such as caffeine and theophylline may be useful in conjunction with ephedrine in enhancing the latter's effect on energy expenditure. Recently, interest has been aroused by a new atypical beta agonist, **BRL 26830A, (455)** which stimulates brown fat thermogenesis in rodents. In one trial this drug enhanced dietary weight loss by 50% with no adverse action other than tremor (ref. 55). Tremor is apparently less of a problem with ICI 198157. Regular injected **growth hormone** which promotes nitrogen retention and increases muscle mass, does not appear to increase weight loss in obese subjects with otherwise normal growth hormone responses. **Alpha-2 adrenergic antagonists** increase lipolysis and thermogenesis through a blockade of the antilipolytic alpha-2-adrenoceptor on fat cell membranes and by activation centrally of the sympathetic nervous system. These compounds, include newer variants (e.g. SK&F 86,466 and RP 55462), are under acute investigation in animals and man.

Table 42. Thermogenic Drugs
• Thyroxine and triiodothyronine
• L dopa
• Ephedrine
• Methyl anthines
• Atypical ß agonist (e.g. BRL 26830A, Ro 40-2148 and ICI 198157)
• Growth hormone
• Alpha-2 adrenergic antagonists (e.g. yohimbine, idazoxan)

Structure of BRL 26830A compared with noradrenaline

Fat Absorption Inhibition

Drugs and dietary preparations which regulate intestinal absorption, especially fat absoption, are under investigation. Such agents include diethylaminoethyl-dextran (DEAE-D), glucosidase inhibitors, dietary fibre and tetrahydrolipstatin. The pharmacological action of **DEAE-D** is similar to that of cholestyramine, binding bile salts in the intestine and hence reducing fat absorption (ref. 56). **Tetrahydrolipstatin** is a selective inhibitor of pancreatic lipase (ref. 57). Weight loss is increased by both agents but side effects such as loose stools, abdominal fullness and flatulence may be a problem in some.

Surgery

Jaw wiring

This is especially useful for rapid weight loss necessary for surgery or ill health. In one large series of 101 patients, wired for 9 months, weight loss averaged 52.6 kg. Regrettably, of the 52 patients followed up after the wires were removed, all regained weight.

Table 43. Operations for Obesity
• Jaw wiring
• Gut bypass
Jejuno-ileal bypass
• Gastric reduction
Gastric bypass
Gastroplasty
• Gastric balloon
• Apronectomy
• Fat suction

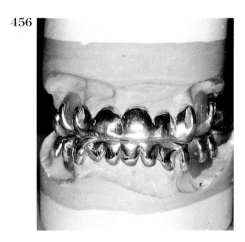

456 Jaw wiring cast. A stainless steel cast is made from a wax impression of the teeth and jaw.

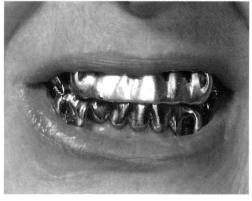

457 Jaw wiring in situ. The steel cast is then cemented to the teeth with wire loops holding the upper and lower jaws together. Liquid food is taken via a straw inserted into a gap in the cast. Two pints of milk with added vitamins provides about 800 kcal (3.4 MJ) per day.

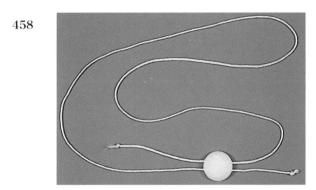

458 Waist cord. To prevent weight regain once the wires are removed Garrow and Gardiner invented a simple device, a waist cord, held in place by a plastic button (ref. 58).

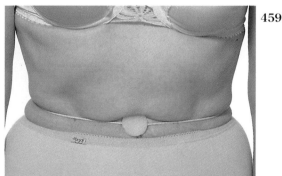

459 Waist cord in situ. Once this patient lost weight the cord was affixed firmly around her waist with the cord ends knotted and held within the plastic button. If the patient gained weight, the extra pressure of the tightened cord was felt as a reminder to eat less.

460

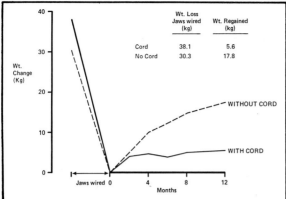

	Wt. Loss Jaws wired (kg)	Wt. Regained (kg)
Cord	38.1	5.6
No Cord	30.3	17.8

460 Weight regain with waist cord. Once jaw wires were removed weight regain over one year was one-third less with a waist cord in position (ref. 58). Waist cords may also be useful in preventing weight regain after dieting. Over an eleven-month follow up, after weight loss on a diet alone, those with a cord lost an additional 4.8 kg, whereas those without regained 6.6 kg (ref. 59). Its use can be limited by a remaining apron of fat, abdominal obesity, patient compliance and acceptability.

Jejuno-ileal bypass and gastroplasty

Before considering surgery certain criteria should be observed:

- Weight either 100% or 45 kg above ideal for 10 years or more.
- Age 18-50 years.
- Absence of a treatable endocrinopathy.
- Failure of supervised non-surgical methods.
- Psychological stability.
- Non-alcoholic.

- Willingness to attend for follow-ups.
- No cardiac ischaemia, renal or liver impairment.
- A disease associated with obesity present such as diabetes mellitus, hyperlipidaemia, arthritis, Pickwickian, hypertension.

The mortality and morbidity is such that most have abandoned jejuno-ileal bypass which is now mainly reserved for severe, medically untreatable hypercholesterolaemia (ref. 60).

461

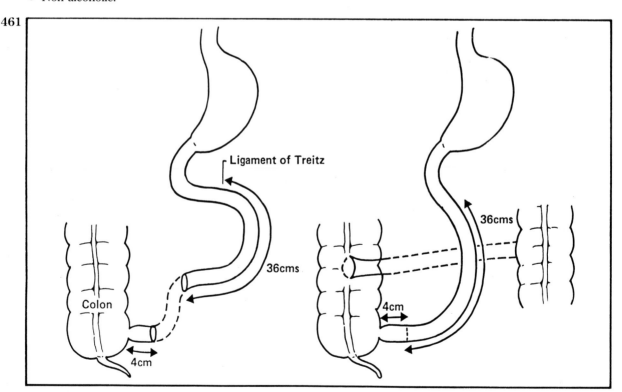

461 Jejuno-ileal bypass. There are many versions of the intestinal bypass operation but a common procedure consists of the removal of the small intestine 36 cm from the ligament of Treitz and 4 cm from the ileocaecal junction. The redundant segment is anastomised with the ascending colon.

Table 44. Complications of jejuno-ileal bypass
Mortality 5%
Morbidity 60-70%
Liver abnormalities 30%
Renal failure 10%
Systemic infections 2-5%
Pancreatitis 1%
Electrolyte and mineral depletion 50% +
Renal calculi 5-20%
Cholelithiasis 10%
Bone disease 50% +
Anorectal disease 50% +
Bypass enteritis 20-50%
Obstruction 5%
Toxic gut dilatation 10-20%
Polyarthralgia 10-15%
Diarrhoea 60%

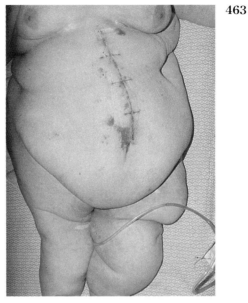

463

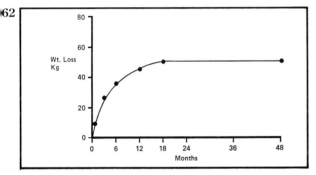

462

462 Weight loss after jejuno-ileal bypass. Weight loss is rapid and substantial but usually levels out after 18 months.

463 Jejuno-ileal bypass after operation. Extensive incision is shown. Often respiratory problems necessitate postoperative ventilation in an intensive therapy unit.

464

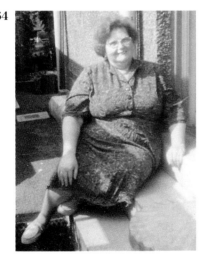

465

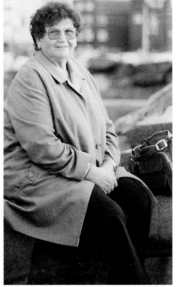

464 & 465 Success after jejuno-ileal bypass. Some patients benefit substantially as did this woman, who lost over 5 stone (32 kg) and regained her self-esteem with jejuno-ileal bypass. **464** shows the patient before the operation and **465** after substantial weight loss.

Roux-en-Y
Gastro-jejunostomy

Disadvantages:
    Technical Difficulty
    Metabolic sequelae

GASTROPLASTY

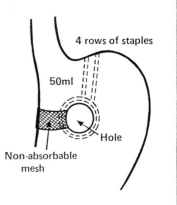

Conditions

1. Proximal pouch 50ml volume at
   25–30 cm of N saline pressure

2. Stoma of 9–12mm diameter

3. Permanent partition with 4 rows
   of staples

4. Reinforcement of the stoma
   with non-absorbable mesh

4 rows of staples

50ml

Hole

Non-absorbable
mesh

466 Gastric bypass. Roux-en-Y gastrojejunostomy.

467 Gastroplasty. There are a number of versions of this operation. In the horizontal banded gastroplasty the line of staples is horizontal and the stoma is at the greater curvature of the stomach. In the vertical banded method (as shown) the line of staples is vertical and the stoma is at the lesser curvature. The vertical method is preferred by many on technical grounds and weight loss does appear to be better than with the horizontal method. Weight loss in a series of 50 patients has been reported to average 26 kg after one year, with no further weight loss thereafter (ref. 61).

Table 45. Complications of Gastroplasty and Gastric Bypass Operations

Mortality 4%
Early — Respiratory failure
           Peritonitis
           Pulmonary embolism
Late — Sudden deaths associated with severe fatty
           liver infiltration

Morbidity 33%
   Nausea and vomiting 10-30%
   Anastomotic leaks, fistulae < 10%
   Dehiscence of staples 5-15%
   Peptic ulcer 2.5%
   Perforation 3%
   Atalectasis 4%
   Malnutrition 2%
   Wound infection 10%
   Hernia 6%
   Cholelithiasis 2-6%

Table 46. Latex Gastric Balloon

Weight Loss:	0.8-1.3 kg/week Balloon vs diet alone: 1.0 vs 0.6-0.7 kg/week
Contra-indications:	Peptic ulcers, hiatus hernia, strictures, potential bleeding lesions
Complications:	3% faint 5% gastric ulceration Epigastric pain, belching, vomiting, nausea, heartburn Intestinal obstruction

---

Gastric balloon

The deflated gastric balloon is inserted into the stomach by gastroscopy and then inflated with air or sterile water to a capacity of up to 500 ml volume. Follow up results with latex balloons have been disappointing. These balloons have a tendency to deflate 7-21 days after insertion. However, McFarland et al have reported that even with an inflated balloon in situ their patients, who lost intially 11 kg in 3 months, regained this weight at the end of one year (ref. 62). Silicone balloons might possibly be more promising as these are more resilient and may have a life span in an inflated state of 3-6 months (ref. 63). Early work with this type of balloon suggests that initial weight loss can be significant, although long term results will be necessary for proper validation. Recent work suggests that silicone, being relatively inert, is associated with fewer complications than latex (**Table 46**).

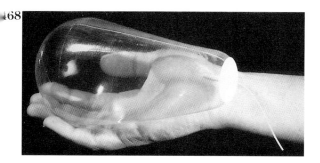

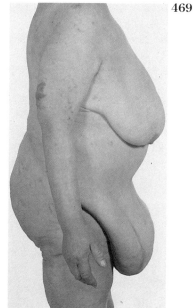

468 Silicone stomach balloon in an inflated state made by Dunlop Precision Rubber. The deflated balloon is inserted into the stomach and inflated to 500 ml with sterile water or Dextran. When it has served its purpose the balloon is punctured and either withdrawn through the oesophagus or passed out through the bowels (ref. 63).

469 Apron of fat is often best dealt with by an apronectomy.

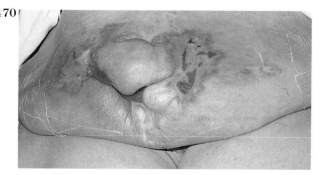

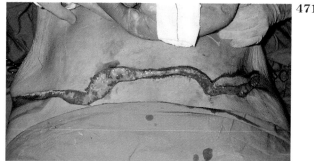

470 Ulceration with infection over apron of fat is a major indication for such an operation.

471 Apronectomy. The apron is lifted upwards and the incision is made below the apron.

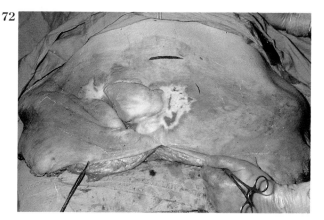

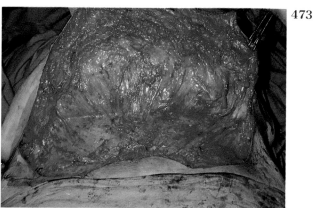

472 Apronectomy — the apron is dissected away.

473 Dissected apron lifted upwards to show the extent of the dissection.

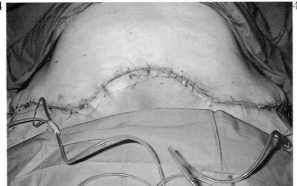

474

474 Apron removed and flaps restitched.

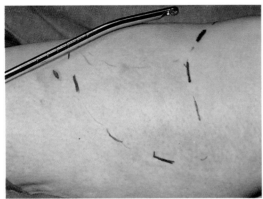

475

475 Fat suction. Suction device is shown. A hyaluronidase solution is injected into the area to be treated.

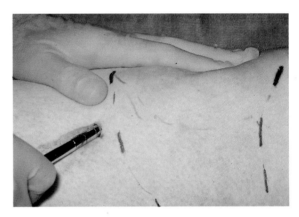

47

476 Fat suction. The suction catheter is inserted subcutaneously and attached to a powerful suction machine. The hand is used here to manoeuvre the fat to achieve a satisfactory cosmetic result.

477

477 Fat removed from an area of lipohypertrophy shown in **475** and **476**. This technique, used by some for removal of large areas of fat, is not without hazard. Free fat is passed into the urine after the operation and fat embolism can occur.

References

1. Obesity: A report of the Royal College of Physicians. Journal of the Royal College of Physicians of London, 1983, 17, 3-58.
2. Garrow JS. Obesity and Related Diseases. Churchill Livingstone, Edinburgh, 1988.
3. Rosenbaum S, Skinner RK, Knight IB and Garrow JS. A survey of heights and weights of adults in Great Britain. Annals of Human Biology 1985, 12, 115-127.
4. Durnin JVGA and Wormersley J. Body fat assessed from total body density and its estimation from skinfold thickness: Measurements on 481 men and women aged 16 to 72 years. British Journal of Nutrition 1974, 32, 77-97.
5. Stunkard AJ, Sorensen TIA, Hanis C, Teasdale TW, Chakraborty R, Schull WJ and Schelsinger F. An adoption study of human obesity. New England Journal of Medicine 1986, 314, 193-198.
6. James WPT, Davies HL, Bailes J and Dauncey MJ. Elevated metabolic rates in obesity. Lancet 1978, 1, 1122-1124.
7. Prentice AM, Black AE, Coward WA, Davies HL, Goldberg GR, Murgatroyd PR, Ashford J, Sawyer M and Whitehead RG. High levels of energy expenditure in obese women. British Medical Journal 1986, 292, 983-987.
8. Morgan JB, York DA, Wasilewska A and Portman J. A study of the thermic responses to a meal and to a sympathomimetic drug (ephedrine) in relation to energy balance in man. British Journal of Nutrition 1982, 47, 21-32.
9. Roberts SB, Savage J, Coward WA, Chew B and Lucas A. Energy expenditure and intake in infants born to lean and overweight mothers. New England Journal of Medicine 1988, 318, 461-466.
10. Geissler CA, Miller DS and Shah M. Daily metabolic rate of the post obese and the lean. American Journal of Clinical Nutrition 1987, 45, 914-920.
11. Ravussen E. Lillioja S, Knowler WC, Christin L, Freymond D, Abbott WGH, Boyce V, Howard BV and Bogardus C. Reduced rate of energy expenditure as a risk factor for body weight gain. New England Journal of Medicine 1988, 318, 467-472.
12. Brooks SL, Rothwell NJ, Stock MJ, Goodbody AE and Trayhurn P. Increased protein conductance pathway in brown adipose tissue mitochondria of rats exhibiting diet induced thermogenesis. Nature 1980, 286, 274-276.
13. Thurlby PL and Trayhurn P. The role of thermoregulatory thermogenesis in the elevated energy of obese (ob/ob) mice pairfed with lean siblings. British Journal of Nutrition 1987, 42, 377-385.
14. Lever JD, Jung RT, Nnodim JO, Leslie PJ and Symons D. Demonstration of a catecholaminergic innervation in human perirenal brown adipose tissue at various ages in the adult. Anatomical Record 1986, 215, 251-255.
15. Norman D, Mukherjee S, Symons D, Jung RT and Lever JD. Neuropeptides in interscapular and perirenal brown adipose tissue in the rat: A plurality of innervation. Journal of Neurocytology 1988, 17, 305-311.
16. Lever JD, Jung RT, Mukherjee S, Norman D, Symons D, Connacher AA and Wheeler MH. Catecholaminergic and peptidergic nerves in naturally occurring and phaeochromocytoma associated brown adipose tissue. Clinical Anatomy, 1989, 2, 157-166.
17. Cunningham S, Leslie P, Hopwood D, Illingworth P, Jung RT, Nicholls DG, Peden N, Rafael J and Rial E. The characterisation and energetic potential of brown adipose tissue in man. Clinical Science 1985, 69, 343-348.
18. Jung RT, Gurr MI, Robinson MP and James WPT. Does adipocyte hypercellularity in obesity exist? British Medical Journal 1978, 2, 319-321.
19. Charney E, Goodman HC, McBridge M, Lyon B and Pratt R. Childhood antecedents of adult obesity. Do chubby infants become obese adults? New England Journal of Medicine 1976, 295, 6-9.

20. Laurance BM, Brito A and Wilkinson J. Prader-Willi syndrome after age 15 years. Archives of Diseases in Childhood 1981, 56, 181-186.
21. Hawkey CJ and Smithies A. The Prader-Willi syndrome with a 15/15 translocation. Journal of Medical Genetics 1976, 13, 152-163.
22. Goldstein JL and Fialkow PJ. The Alström syndrome. Report of three cases with further delineation of the clinical, pathophysiological and genetic aspects of the disorder. Medicine 1973, 52, 53-71.
23. Goecke T, Majewski F. Kauther KD and Sterzel U. Mental retardation, hypotonia, obesity, ocular, facial, dental and limb abnormality (Cohen syndrome). European Journal of Paediatrics 1982, 138, 338-340.
24. The New Medicine: An integrated system of study, Volume 2, 'Endocrinology'. Editors: Hart I and Newton R. MTP Press, London, England, 1984.
25. Leslie P, Jung RT, Baty R, Newton RW, Isles T and Illingworth P. The effect of optimal glycaemic control with continuous subcutaneous insulin infusion in energy expenditure in Type I diabetes mellitus. British Medical Journal 1986, 293, 1121-1126.
26. Thompson C and White MC. A case of insulinoma. In series Endocrinology Casebook. Editors: Jung RT and Chahal P. Hospital Update 1987, 13, 538-548.
27. Lew EA and Garfinkel L. Variations in mortality by weight among 750,000 men and women. Journal of Chronic Diseases 1979, 32, 563-576.
28. Rimm AA, Werner LH, Van Yserloo B and Bernstein RA, Relationship of obesity and disease in 73,532 weight-conscious women. Public Health Reports 1975, 90, 44-51.
29. Tuck ML, Sowers J, Dornfeld L Kledzik G and Maxwell M. Effect of weight reduction on blood pressure, plasma renin activity and plasma aldosterone levels in obese patients. New England Journal of Medicine 1981, 304, 930-933.
30. Chalmers N and Campbell I. Phlegmasia coerulia dolens revisited. The Practitioner 1987, 231, 1519-1521.
31. Reid JM, Fullmer SD, Pettigrew KD, Burch TA, Bennett PM, Miller M and Wheldon GD. Nutrient intake of Pima women: Relationship to diabetes mellitus and gallstone disease. American Journal of Clinical Nutrition 1971, 24, 1281-1289.
32. Friedman GD, Kannel WB and Dawber TR. The epidemiology of gallbladder disease: Observations in the Framingham Study. Journal of Chronic Diseases 1966, 19, 273-292.
33. Duncan ID. Advances in the prevention and treatment of gynaecological malignancy. Update 1986, 33, 775-784.
34. Bray GA. Complications of obesity. Annals of Internal Medicine 1985, 103, 1052-1061.
35. Dunaif A, Graf M, Mandeli J, Laumas V and Dobrjansky A. Characterisation of groups of hyperandrogenic women with acanthosis nigricans, impaired glucose tolerance and/or hyperinsulinaemia. Journal of Clinical Endocrinology and Metabolism 1987, 65, 499-507.
36. Stuart CA, Peters EJ, Prince MJ, Richard G, Cavallo A and Meyer WJ. Insulin resistance with acanthosis nigricans: The role of obesity and androgen excess. Metabolism 1986, 35, 197-205.
37. Matsuoka LY, Wortsman J, Gavin JR and Goldmann J. Spectrum of endocrine abnormalities associated with acanthosis nigricans. American Jounral of Medicine 1987, 83, 719-725.
38. Westlund K and Nicolayson R. A ten year mortality and morbidity related to serum cholesterol. A follow-up of 3751 men aged 40-49. Scandinavian Journal of Laboratory Investigation 1972, 30, Suppl. 127, 1-24.
39. Nuttall FQ. Gynaecomastia as a physical finding in normal men. Journal of Clinical Endocrinology and Metabolism 1979, 48, 338-340.

40. Dexter CJ. Benign enlargement of the male breast. New England Journal of Medicine 1956, 254, 996-997.

41. Williams Textbook of Endocrinology, 7th Edition. Editors: Wilson JD and Foster DW. Saunders Co., 1985. Endocrine Disorders of the Breast: Frantz AG and Wilson JD, p410-416.

42. Kalkhoff R and Ferrow C. Metabolic differences between obese, overweight and muscular overweight. New England Journal of Medicine 1971, 284, 1236-1239.

43. Williams T. Berelowitz M, Joffe SN, Thorner MO, Rivier J, Vale W and Frohman LA. Impaired growth hormone responses to growth hormone releasing factor in obesity. New England Journal of Medicine 1984, 311, 1403-1407.

44. Amatruda JM, Hochstein M, Hsu T-H and Lockwood DH. Hypothalamic and pituitary dysfunction in obese males. International Journal of Obesity 1982, 6, 183-189.

45. Jung RT. Endocrinological aspects of obesity. Clinics in Endocrinology and Metabolism 1984, 13, 597-612.

46. Jung RT, Campbell RG, James WPT and Callingham BA. Altered hypothalamic and sympathetic responses to hypoglycaemia in familial obesity. Lancet 1982, i, 1043-1046.

47. Kopelman PG. Neuroendocrine function in obesity. Clinical Endocrinology 1988, 28, 675-689.

48. Kley HK, Solbarch HG, McKinnan JC and Krushemper HL. Testosterone decrease and oestrogen increase in male patients with obesity. Acta Endocrinolgica 1979, 91, 553-563.

49. Kopelman PG. Clinical complications of obesity. Clinics in Endocrinology and Metabolism 1984, 13, 613-634.

50. Douglas NJ. Breathing during sleep in adults. Recent Advances in Respiratory Medicine, Chapter 14, 1988, p231-248. Churchill Livingstone, Edinburgh.

51. Cohen AH. Massive obesity and the kidney. American Journal of Pathology 1975, 81, 117-130.

52. Warnke A and Kempson RL. Nephrotic syndrome in massive obesity. Archives of Pathology and Laboratory Medicine 1978, 102, 431-438.

53. Stunkard AJ, Craighead LW and O'Brien R. The treatment of obesity: A controlled trial of behaviour therapy, pharmacotherapy and their combination. Lancet 1980, i, 1045-1047.

54. Astrup A, Lundsgaard C, Madsen J and Christensen NJ. Enhanced thermogenic responsiveness during chronic ephedrine treatment in man. American Journal of Clinical Nutrition 1985, 42, 83-94.

55. Connacher AA, Jung RT and Mitchell PEG. Increased weight loss in diet restricted obese subjects given BRL 26830A — A new atypical ß agonist. British Medical Journal 1988, 296, 1217-1220.

56. Cairella M. Use of DEAE-D in the treatment of obesity. International Journal of Obesity 1987, 11, Supplement 3, 225-227.

57. Hogan S, Fleury A, Hadvary P, Lengsfeld H. Meier MK, Triscari J and Sullivan AC. Studies on the antiobesity activity of tetrahydrolipstatin, a potent and selective inhibitor of pancreatic lipase. International Journal of Obesity 1987, 11, Supplement 3, 35-42.

58. Garrow JS and Gardiner GT. Maintenance of weight loss in obese patients after jaw wiring. British Medical Journal 1981, 282, 858-860.

59. Simpson GK, Farquhar DL, Carr P, Galloway S McL, Stewart IC, Donald P, Steven F and Munro JF. Intermittent protein sparing fasting with abdominal belting. International Journal of Obesity 1986, 10, 247-254.

60. Holt PR and Kotler DP. Surgical Management of morbid obesity and hyperlipidaemia. In Diabetes Mellitus and Obesity. Chapter 37. Editors: Brodoff BN, Bleicher SJ. Williams and Wilkins, Baltimore and London, 1982, pp333-340.

61. Anderson T, Backer OG, Stokholm KH and Quaade F. Randomised trial of diet and gastroplasty for morbid obesity. New England Journal of Medicine 1984, 310, 352-356.

62. McFarland RJ, Grundy A, Gazet JC and Pilkington TRE. The intragastric balloon: A novel idea proved ineffective. British Journal of Surgery 1987, 74, 137-139.

63. Durrans D, Taylor TV, Pullan BR and Rose P. Intragastric balloons. Journal of the Royal College of Surgeons of Edinburgh 1985, 30, 369-371.

Index (Figures refer to page numbers)